FIT
AND
HEALTHY
THROUGHOUT
LIFE

TRACY DWYER

GLASS**SPIDER**PUBLISHING

Cover design by Judith S. Design & Creativity
www.judithsdesign.com
Published by Glass Spider Publishing
www.glassspiderpublishing.com

To Isabella, Alexandra, and Evangelina.

Contents

Chapter 1: Your Attitude Determines Your Outcome

Do you ever look at people who are in shape and wish you knew their secrets? Do you see people who eat healthy and wish you had the willpower to do the same? Do you ever see an athlete and wish you were able to do what they do? What would you try if you knew you would not fail?

I can tell you from personal experience that you can achieve whatever you believe you can do. Your internal voice provides inspiration, and the physical method of articulating the idea by writing it down is the first step to realization. This is a great way to get yourself into the frame of mind to be successful. All the things that you know you can achieve, you will achieve.

If you procrastinate and continually feel that someday you may be able to try to do something to get into shape, you are already planting the seeds of disappointment and possible failure in your mind. By using positive mantras and visualizing yourself being successful at doing the things you want to do in your life, you will be able to achieve them. By training your brain for success and not letting negative thoughts enter your mind, this new program installed in your brain will propel you toward your goals.

Your brain is a very complicated machine, yet it is also very simplistic in its desires and needs. The brain requires protein to build neurotransmitters, called message transmitters, that help brain cells communicate. The brain needs carbohydrates from whole foods such as legumes, beans, fruits, and vegetables for high-quality fuel for brain function. The carbohydrates are broken down into glucose to be used by the brain for cell activity. The brain needs water to stay hydrated. If the brain loses too much water, it will not work efficiently.

The brain also needs stimulation from the outside world as well as the inside world. Besides eating whole foods and having a healthy eating plan, you also need to have positive self-talk. Positive self-talk is vital to success. If you believe that you will be successful at whatever you want to do, you are much closer to achieving your goals.

Books like the Bible, *As a Man Thinketh*, and more are about believing in yourself and how this relates to what you become. Act as if you already have what you want, and talk to yourself as though you already are the person you want to be. This is very powerful. Thinking this way will bring your goals to reality. If you constantly tell yourself that you are a failure, cannot eat healthy, cannot lose weight, hate to exercise, cannot get up early, don't have time to eat healthy or exercise, it will plant the seed of doubt and failure in your mind.

Success is made by believing you can achieve your goals. Changing the way you communicate with yourself is a very powerful way of becoming the person you want to be. Loving yourself will make you more loveable and attractive to others. It will make you more powerful, and it will attract people who are like-minded. You don't want to attract negative people who are always down on themselves. You want strong, powerful people around you who are the "movers and shakers" of the world.

Where are the groups of people who have the same goal in mind? They are supportive, positive, and will help you focus on the goal. They are groups of people who have the same goal in mind, whether it's to get on my healthy eating plan, be a healthier person, start an exercise program, start hiking, biking, running, going to the gym, or any positive activity you want to do. Being around like-minded, positive people will bring about a positive way of thinking that will lead to your goals being realized. When you put yourself in the state of mind to be successful, you will be successful. Putting your health as the number-one priority and knowing you will succeed at being healthy is what will make your goals a reality.

Negative thoughts and words can keep you from realizing your dream and moving forward in life, and they can make you physically ill. When you have negative thoughts or feelings, write them down on a piece of paper and throw them in the trash. This is a good way to let your mind know that you're done with negative thoughts. This can be done with your negative self-talk as well as anyone in your life who is keeping you down or holding you back. Negative thoughts and people are toxic and don't belong in your life. Realize what's holding you back or making you feel like you're not worthy and get rid of them, just like the paper you threw in the trash.

Years ago, I went to a very informative seminar that demonstrated just how negative thoughts prevent positive outcomes. In the beginning, everyone was given a wooden board that was the size of a book. We were instructed to write on the board four things we could have in life if nothing was holding us back. Then on the other side, we were asked to write four things that were stopping us from attaining the things we want in life.

During the seminar, we learned how to conquer those negative thoughts to prevent them from holding us back. At the end, we lined up in groups and each person gave their piece of wood to the people in front. We were instructed to hold the negative side of the board toward us and use the palm of our hand to break the board in half to symbolize nothing was going to hold us back in life. We were told to visualize breaking through the board without any doubts in our minds.

One by one, people broke through that strong piece of wood. When it was my turn, I started out confidently but then worried I would hurt my hand. That second of doubt kept me from breaking the board. The instructors said to visualize yourself breaking the board and not to take your focus off being successful and getting everything you want in life. The thought was planted deep in my mind, and I hit the board as hard as I could and smashed through the wood, breaking it in half.

I was filled with joy and power, knowing I could train my mind that quickly to overcome fear. To this day, I have that broken board sitting on my desk to remind myself of how strong I am. Everything on the back of that board I have achieved in my life, proving what a powerful tool the mind is. The mind can be filled with positive thoughts that can propel you to achieve many things if you use it wisely. Exercise your mind daily by using positive words and thoughts all day and night.

There are many things that we think during the day and night, and all those thoughts affect who we are and how we react to things. People who believe that everything is going to go well and that things always work out will experience more positive outcomes in life. People who feel they're unlucky or that bad things always happen to them usually experience negative things in life. It is a known fact that our thoughts affect who we are and how we react to things, but they also affect how we experience things. People with a positive outlook will see situations as positive. People with a negative outlook on life will experience negativity.

Have you ever looked outside and seen a cloudy sky and thought that it might rain, making it a bad day? Have you been with a person who looks at the same sky and always finds something beautiful about the it even if it's dark and gloomy? Those are the people who experience positive things in their life. The people who look at life as a beautiful adventure will find joy in life. People who always complain and look at the negative things in life set themselves up to fail or not experience progress.

We never know what's going to happen in life, but if we expect great things to happen, they will. There's something about being a positive person that makes every minute of every day special. Feeling happy inside and showing it on the outside with your face, smile, body posture, and language makes living each day a wonderful experience. Isn't it better to feel healthy every day than to feel tired, depressed, anxious, and lifeless?

Think of something in life that you really want to happen. Close your eyes and imagine it happening. Notice how you feel at that moment, and feel all the joyous emotions of success and happiness. Take the same situation and just hope that it's going to go right, and see how your posture, facial expressions, and thoughts change. Even though nothing has happened yet, there's still a big change when you just hope something is going to happen instead of thinking that it is going to happen. This is how much our thoughts affect our lives.

Like everyone, I've had bad experiences but always thought I was going to get through them and be successful. I got a full scholarship to my dream school, Pepperdine University in Malibu, as a pre-med student. Through hard work, I was determined to earn a full scholarship, and I did just that.

When I was 36, I was diagnosed with colon cancer and had to put my power of positive thinking to work. I pictured myself being cured of cancer. I repeated my mantra of happily and joyfully being cured of cancer and not requiring any further treatment over and over, all day long. After the surgery, the doctor did a biopsy on the 10 inches of my colon that he took out and said the cancer had not spread and I would require no further treatment.

A good way to be successful is to imagine yourself being successful and never thinking that you're going to fail. When starting off with this high expectation, you will be successful. Condition yourself to always act like you already have what you want in life. Walk and talk like you're successful, and never utter a negative word. Always look for the positive in everything you do. You'll notice that life goes in the right direction, and you become the successful person you want to be.

This way of thinking can be used in every area of your life to achieve whatever you want. If you want to meet the man or woman of your dreams, make sure you know what that person is like and be very specific. If you want a partner that is active, fit, successful, educated, professional, has a good career, is good looking, has a good sense of humor, and whatever else you can think of, make a list and stick to it. Know that you're going to meet a person who is perfect for you, and don't settle for anything less.

I added to my list that I wanted someone who would love me unconditionally. After I wrote down my list and said it out loud, I asked God to send me this man. Two months later, I met my husband, and he is all that and more. When I wanted to be an actor, I had a mantra which was, "I am happily acting in television, movies, and commercials." I took some acting classes and headshots and signed on with an agent, and my phone started to ring. I was called to do acting jobs on television, in movies, and in commercials. I know firsthand how powerful words, thoughts, and mantras are and how the power of positive thinking can get you what you want and where you want to be in life.

What is success, and how do you become successful in life? The answer to that question depends on who you are and what you want from life. One person's idea of success may be to make a million dollars or to climb to the top of a mountain. Each person must measure their own success in life.

When you look at your life, do you feel good about yourself? Do you feel you've succeeded in the game of life? Some people would say yes because they continue to move forward no matter what happens. Others would say no because they haven't achieved their one big goal, which is to hike to the top of a mountain or run a marathon.

Many people talk about success in the area of weight loss. Someone who has lost weight and kept the weight off will feel successful. Someone who has been trying to lose weight for years and hasn't achieved that goal will most likely feel unsuccessful.

Weight loss can be achieved by following a healthy eating plan, such as the one I outline in my book *Healthy Meals in Minutes*. By eating healthy meals and getting daily exercise, you will lose weight and be able to keep the weight off. Your success can be measured in your ability to stick with the plan, which will improve your health and help you lose weight. Don't wait until you've lost all the weight you want or need to lose to feel successful. Starting the journey to good health begins today, and once you start, you will be successful.

Everything I've learned throughout my life and in my education has brought me to the point I'm at today. My healthy eating plan has worked for me and many other people. I've been able to maintain my weight, physical strength, stamina, brainpower, and health while experiencing the highs and lows that come from living life. I practice what I teach and have learned that everyone can attain the same health I enjoy.

By eating all the necessary food groups in their natural state, the body gets all the nutrients it needs to stay healthy. By enjoying my healthy eating plan, getting regular exercise, and passing along this important information to your family and others, you can be the person you have longed to be.

Chapter 2: Lose Weight, Eat Great

I'm sure this isn't the first book you've bought in an effort to lose weight and live a healthy lifestyle. Many of you have gone on a diet that you heard about, and it may have worked at first, but you got tired of eating the required foods, or not eating carbohydrates, or trying to find gluten-free foods.

A diet with grains, legumes, yams, squash, potatoes, and fruit, along with 100% whole grains, gives your body all the energy and brainpower it needs. These foods also give your body the vital fiber it needs to keep you feeling full and aid in the elimination process. Forget the candy, pastries, white flour products, sugary drinks, soft drinks, toppings, condiments, and sauces with high-fructose corn syrup, sugar, bad fats, and artificial color and flavor. They are bad for your health. By cutting out sugary drinks, candy, soft drinks, high-sugar condiments, and high-fructose corn syrup, you will be eating foods that are full of nutrients.

Many have tried fad diets that are both high in fat and low in fiber and vital nutrients the body needs. Other fads that require pills or claim to reduce fat in certain areas, or intermittent fasting, which is going long periods of time without eating, don't work. The problem with most of these fad diets is they're typically too hard to maintain and are not healthy. Cutting out food groups, especially carbohydrates that feed the brain, affects your health in negative ways. Choose to be healthy and eat foods the way they were intended to be eaten, and enjoy the taste of real food.

What you need to know about fad diets
Many diets sound promising and offer fast results, but they're usually not good for you. Most men need a minimum of 2,500 calories a day to sustain metabolism, muscle activity, and brain function. Most women need 2,000 calories a day. The number varies between age groups, activity levels, and gender. Regardless of who you are, if you eat too many calories, you'll gain weight, which can lead to a variety of diseases. Your body runs on protein, carbohydrates, and fat. By eating foods in their natural states, such as fruits, vegetables, lean protein, 100% whole grains, and healthy fats, your body will be getting the nutrients it needs to stay healthy. Fad diets such as Paleo, Atkins, Keto, and services such as premade meals delivered to your door, intermittent fasting, and other diets, tend to ignore these facts.

Paleo and Atkins diets
The trainer from *The Biggest Loser*, Bob Harper, wrote a book and went on talk shows talking about how great the Paleo diet is. He had a heart attack and almost died. He then went on a talk show and wrote another book about how the body needs healthy carbohydrates and the Paleo diet is too high in fat. Now he is advertising a drug to prevent him from having another heart attack.

The Paleo diet is promoted to improve gut health, but it causes a shift in gut microbiota composition along with increased serum trimethylamine-N-oxide (TMAO) levels. Paleo focuses on consuming high-protein meat, fish, eggs, seeds, nuts, and low-carbohydrate vegetables and fruit, and eliminates dairy, all grains, legumes including peanut butter, and refined and processed foods. The typical Paleo diet puts you at risk for deficiencies in calcium and vitamin D which is critical to bone health. The Paleo diet also includes saturated fat and protein being consumed far above recommended levels increasing the risk of kidney, heart disease, and certain types of cancer.

Eating a diet that is high in fat and protein with little or no healthy carbohydrates is not a healthy diet. This type of diet puts a lot of stress on your body and digestive system. This diet without fiber, or very little fiber, causes constipation, which is another stress on the body. This diet also is void of the nutrients you get from fruits and vegetables, which are vital for good health, leaving people craving carbohydrates because the body needs healthy carbohydrates.

Protein helps to build muscle and bone but does not have the vital nutrients, vitamins, and fiber your body needs to fight diseases. Fruits and vegetables also help you feel full and satisfied for a long period. When you eat 100% whole grains like brown rice, oats, and quinoa, which has protein and fiber, your meals will be satisfying and keep you from craving sugar and junk foods. Recognize that just because a celebrity on an advertisement being paid to say the fad diet helped them lose weight doesn't mean it's healthy for the body.

Keto diet
The Atkins diet is another fad diet that overindulges in high fat and red meats and limits the healthy complex carbohydrates necessary for overall health. Keto is another type of low-carbohydrate diet,

but it leans on the stricter side of low carb with high-fat bacon, avocados, and butter to maintain a rigid nutritional plan where the body goes into ketosis. This is a process the body goes into when it's not getting enough carbohydrates for energy. The body will start to use fat for energy but will also use muscle when not enough carbohydrates are available.

Ketosis is the state the body goes into when it thinks it's starving. The 10 signs of ketosis are bad breath, increased ketones in the blood, increased ketones in the breath or urine, lack of energy, suppressed appetite, fatigue, and decrease in performance. Promoters of this diet will say that is short-term but depends on the individual and activity level.

The weight loss will initially be in the form of water weight due to lack of fiber and loss of muscle mass due to lack of carbohydrates for energy. The brain also runs on carbohydrates, so brain fog is one of the side effects of low-carbohydrate diets. This low-carbohydrate diet also causes constipation since fiber is needed to aid the elimination process. The term "keto flu" refers to symptoms people experience within ketosis such as headache, tiredness, nausea, and stomach upset.

Testing the blood and urine is the best way to know if you're in ketosis, but the smell and symptoms will also let you know. A diet that causes the body to go into ketosis, making the body think it's starving, will make the body consume anything, including muscle, to function. This can be very dangerous, and the high fat in the diet is unhealthy and lacks vital nutrients everybody needs.

Spot reduction
Many people worry about unwanted belly fat and try to find ways to reduce it. There are many advertisements for supplements that are supposed to target and reduce belly fat at a very fast rate. These

supplements have a variety of ingredients such as stimulants that are said to melt the belly fat away. Targeting belly fat or spot reducing a single part of the body is a difficult thing to do. Belly fat can be part of your genetic makeup, or it can be caused by stress that raises the cortisol hormone in your body, or excessive alcohol consumption and can lead to weight gain around your midsection.

Packaged mean plans

Premade meal services are usually expensive, restrictive, and not a good option for those who are on a budget. They are typically sent to your home in small portions that limit calories while you adhere to their meal plans. For those who like to choose their own meals and prepare them fresh, the options are very limited. The meals are extremely small for the price, and there is a lot of pasta on the sample menu.

A typical sample menu would include breakfast of a double chocolate muffin, low-fat plain yogurt, and coffee. The morning snack is a small bag of almonds. Lunch is white cheddar macaroni and cheese with green salad, and the afternoon snack is strawberries and string cheese. Dinner is chicken and pasta with broccoli, and a small snickerdoodle cookie for dessert. There are options for a diabetes plan, which you can look up if you like.

The point is you can do all this yourself, buying the proper foods at the grocery store and having healthier meals that you can prepare in minutes. Buy my book *Healthy Meals in Minutes*, where I show you how to choose the right foods and navigate the grocery store so you don't end up with junk foods and unhealthy snacks. Learn how to prepare your own meals and how to cook delicious meals in minutes for yourself and your family.

The most important thing to remember when you want to lose weight and stay healthy is to stay on a healthy eating plan. The key is keeping your blood sugar stable by eating foods that are in their natural state, high in fiber and nutritional value, and stopping eating junk foods. Avoid fad diets that cut out vital nutrients, especially complex carbohydrates which are vital to good health and brain function. These new fad diets are high in fat and calories.

On low-calorie diets, you will lose weight, but it will be from a loss of muscle mass and water weight. The body needs enough calories to function. Your body is constantly using calories even when you're sleeping. During sleep is when your body is repairing itself and regenerating. A 125-pound person will burn approximately 38 calories an hour and sleep seven to nine hours a night, which will be 266-342 calories burned while asleep. The more muscle you have, the more calories you burn through the day and at night.

Chapter 3: Main Causes of Weight Gain and How to Eliminate Them

There are many reasons why people gain weight, and many of the main causes can be controlled. The most common reasons are sugary foods and beverages, highly processed foods, alcohol, trans fat, high fat or low protein diet, fruit juice, wrong gut bacteria, inactivity, eating large amounts of food or overeating, stress, and certain medications.

Sugar

Consuming sugary snacks and energy or caffeine drinks loaded with flavorings, whipped cream, caramel, or just adding sugar to your beverage increases the amount of sugar and the associated calories. Processed foods have a lot of fat, sugar, and artificial ingredients. Empty calories that are in sugary drinks, candy, and pastries all spike your blood sugar and leave you craving more food and sugary snacks where you're stuck in an endless cycle of eating and trying to keep energy levels up. When blood sugar drops, it makes you feel sleepy and willing to eat anything that will make you feel good and more energetic. This is how many people pack on the pounds.

Sugary drinks and high-fructose corn syrup (HFCS) are the cause of many problems such as obesity, diabetes, and a higher risk of heart disease. According to the Harvard T. H. Chan School of Public Health, people who drink one to two sugary drinks a day have a 26% greater chance of developing type 2 diabetes than those who rarely drink sugary drinks. For example, a Monster Energy drink has 110 calories per serving, and it has two servings, which makes it 220 calories. The Monster Energy drink has 27 grams of sugar and 80 milligrams of caffeine per eight ounces. The Monster Mega has 240 milligrams of caffeine and 81 grams of sugar. As a comparison, eight ounces of coffee has 94.7 milligrams of caffeine and no sugar.

Caffeine is not recommended for teenagers or children because it's harmful to the nervous system and causes sleeping problems. The amount of caffeine, sugar, and calories are excessive and should be avoided by children, teens, and adults. Keep in mind that the labeling reflects the amount per serving, making the actual amount for the whole can double or in some cases triple if the serving size is three. These caffeinated drinks have other stimulants in them that when combined with caffeine can affect the heart and cause behavior and sleep problems. They provide no nutritional value, cause weight gain, and should be avoided.

Your body will let you know what it needs if you just listen to it and get away from fast foods and junk foods that are loaded with sugar, unhealthy fats, and sodium. When you acquire a taste for salt and sugar, it becomes a craving. Salt and sugar are both acquired tastes. If you never ate them, you wouldn't crave them, and when you stop eating them, you'll stop craving them. When you aren't eating salt and sugar, you'll be able to taste the flavor of fruits and vegetables and 100% whole grains, brown rice, and quinoa. You'll start to crave those foods instead of junk foods. It may take a week or two for the cravings to go away, but if you give your body the nutrients it needs, you'll be able to understand the cravings are for complex carbohydrates, legumes, and lean proteins.

Sugar substitutes such as stevia leaf and xylitol can also assist with weight loss. Stevia leaf has no calories and is all-natural. Xylitol and erythritol are classified as sugar alcohols that have been approved for use in food products in the United States and other parts of the world. There are about 1/3 fewer calories in xylitol than sugar, and it does not promote tooth decay. It was discovered by a Scottish chemist, John Stenhouse, in 1848. It's found in small amounts in plants and fruits such as pears, watermelon, mushrooms, grapes, wine, soy sauce, and sake. It can be used by diabetics and those following a low-carbohydrate diet. It does not spike blood sugar the way table sugar does. When consumed in large amounts, it can cause stomachaches, headaches, and even diarrhea in some people. It is very sweet, which means you can use less to avoid these problems if you're sensitive. Check the label of low calorie or no added sugar products to see if they contain alcoholic sugars such as erythritol. Gum and candy may also contain sugar alcohols.

Alcohol

Drinking alcohol has a double gut punch because it slows down your metabolism and adds a lot of empty calories. These drinks have extra ingredients like syrups, liqueurs, whipped cream, and mixes that add more flavors, sugar, and calories. A margarita has about 230 calories with just one shot of alcohol. If you get a double shot, it adds about 60 more calories, and the calories add up fast. Alcohol also increases appetite due to the impairment of judgment and the fact that it makes you less conscious of what you're eating. This, combined with slowing down the metabolism, makes it easy to see how drinking alcohol causes weight gain. This doesn't mean you can't have an occasional glass of wine, but be aware that it adds about 225 calories, and red wine has even more calories and sugar.

The daily calorie count can add up very fast when you drink alcohol, leading to weight gain. Also, drinking more than one glass of alcohol a day increases your chance of getting cancer in addition to weight gain around the midsection like a beer gut. Women who drink one glass of any type of alcohol every day, even red wine, have a 9% higher risk of getting breast cancer or another type of cancer than those who drink less or not at all. Men are at 5% higher risk of cancer if they drink more than two alcoholic beverages a day.

There have been reports made that say drinking one to two glasses of red wine a day has health benefits. I've read many studies and know many people who are fit and active and love life without alcohol. You don't need alcohol to have a good time or to relax. Alcohol doesn't help you sleep, either, as it interrupts normal sleep patterns. Alcohol may help you fall asleep faster, but it reduces the quality of sleep. Alcohol consumption is studied by many and researched to find out if there are any benefits to drinking alcohol. Several studies mention that alcohol reduces sleep latency at all doses. You'll fall asleep faster and sleep deeper primarily when body repairs, but you are more likely to disrupt the sleep cycle, which changes from rapid eye movement (REM) and non-rapid eye movement, which the body changes approximately every 90 minutes. Non-REM sleep is important for your brain and the repair of tissue, bones, and muscle strength.

Alcohol may help you sleep deeply at first, but it will likely cause you to wake up and be more restless during the second part of the night. Alcohol disrupts the required normal cycle of sleep. Does this mean you should never have a drink? That is an option, but if you have an occasional drink and aren't drinking and driving, it would probably be okay—but in the long run, daily alcohol consumption is not good for your sleep or for your body to repair and grow.

Another place where alcohol will affect your body is in your weight loss and maintaining a sleek, muscular figure. Alcohol goes straight to the gut and can also be seen in the gluteus of women. Many people lose weight but continue to drink alcohol daily, and their body retains the alcohol in areas or causes weight gain around the abdomen. If you want ripped abs, stay away from alcohol. If you drink something once or twice a month that is low in sugar and calories like vodka and tonic, it would most likely not affect you.

Alcohol adds a lot of unnecessary calories and isn't good for your health. Choose not to drink alcohol and encourage your kids, no matter how old they are, to live an alcohol-free life. If you're celebrating a special occasion and have a glass of wine or champagne, it will still add about 200 extra calories to your calorie count for the day, but an occasional drink won't harm your health if you aren't driving and you don't make it a habit.

When alcohol becomes a habit, it will put on extra pounds, especially around the abdomen, and it can contribute to many health issues if you continue drinking regularly. If you're having challenges, there are holistic practitioners, like acupuncturists, that can help you quit drinking if you're using alcohol to relax. If you think alcohol helps you sleep, it's not true. Alcohol keeps you from getting a good and restorative night's sleep. It may make you feel sleepy, but it doesn't help you sleep.

Drinking water is the best way to replenish electrolytes and hydrate your body. When you're dehydrated, you will feel hungry. By drinking a lot of water, your body will stay hydrated and you won't get those food cravings caused by dehydration. Dehydration can cause you to feel dizzy and make you feel lightheaded. Make sure to drink a lot of water to avoid these problems. For something special, have sparkling water with lime, lemon, or a splash of juice on the rocks.

This was always my favorite drink when I went out with friends. It kept people from asking me why I wasn't drinking or asking if they could buy me a drink. I don't need to drink alcohol and don't feel I'm missing out on anything except the extra calories. My health is the most important aspect of my life. My day starts with a big glass of water when I wake up, and I drink a big bottle of water when I work out. I always carry water with me and drink it throughout the day. Water carries nutrients and oxygen to your cells and helps the immune system fight off infection. This calorie-free drink is essential for the body.

Stress

Gaining weight can be caused by stress, which raises the cortisol hormone in your body and can lead to weight gain around your midsection. Stress is part of our daily lives no matter what time of year it is, but how you handle it will determine how productive you are when facing additional stress.

If you are a person who is easy-going and flexible, stress can be productive and even motivate you to do more without getting overwhelmed. Feeling overwhelmed is an emotion that can drag you down if you let it. When you get overwhelmed, it can cause you to get angry, tired, or very wound up and unable to relax or sleep. Turning down the noise in your head will become a constant struggle and may lead to feeling sick or unable to function. For this reason, you need to take the word and the feeling of being overwhelmed out of your mind and vocabulary.

Stress is one of the worst things that we deal with daily. Stress can cause illness and can even cause death if you let it get the best of you. Everyone has stress to a certain degree, and many people don't realize how much it affects their health. Stress can make your blood pressure and heart rate go up and keep you from sleeping at night. If you learn to deal with your stress in a healthy way, it can be motivating and not damaging.

A good example is a stack of books or papers on your desk that you need to go through. Many people would get mad about having so much extra work to do and take more time stressing or complaining about how much work they have instead of just taking a section at a time and handling it. It takes more time to complain about something than it does to handle it. The way to handle it is to do one task at a time. Don't try to tackle the entire mess at one time. Instead of being overwhelmed by the whole mountain of work you must do, just take one piece and handle it. Once you handle one thing, the next will become easier to do. By breaking the mountain down into smaller piles, it's easier to handle.

Stress reduction can also be achieved by changing your perception of situations in your life. If you put two people in the exact same situation with the same amount of stress, one person may get upset and react violently while the other will remain calm without letting the stress get to them. If you let everything that happens in your life get you upset, it will start to wear you down and make you less able to handle pressure and stress.

Practice being calm, and look at situations as challenging or a call to act instead of letting the situation control you and get you upset. It's not good for the heart or the mind to get upset over things in your life. The more times you handle stressful situations by remaining calm, the easier it will be for you to stay in control. The more you overreact and get upset, the more this negative pattern occurs and the less productive you'll become. It's a matter of looking at life or a particular situation with a "glass half full" approach and seeing the positive parts of the situation or how you can make it a positive situation. When your glass is always half full, you have a positive outlook on life. The negative will be replaced with positive, and you will become a very optimistic person.

When I have many tasks to do and some are all-consuming, I find that it's best not to look at the big picture or project and how long it's going to take to get it done. I look at a small piece or task of the project and see how long I can commit to just that part of the project in one day. Breaking it down to how many hours I can spend writing has enabled me to take a very time-consuming task and get it done over time. Instead of putting a stressful timeline on writing a book and how long it will take me to get to a completed manuscript, I set a certain number of hours each day that I will commit to my writing.

My husband says, "How do you eat an elephant? You eat it one forkful at a time." He is great at taking very large tasks and breaking them down into manageable pieces so he makes progress each day and doesn't get stressed out. This is a helpful way to deal with everything in life. Break it down to manageable pieces and do a little each day.

During stressful times, it's easy to gain weight because stress causes your cortisol levels to go up. Cortisol is a hormone that causes you to gain body fat and can contribute to belly fat. The best way to keep your cortisol levels under control is to manage your stress by finding ways to keep yourself calm. This is much harder than it seems until you use techniques that actually lower your heart rate, like deep breathing, meditation, and guided imagery. Activities like exercise, yoga, Pilates, and dancing also help keep your cortisol levels down and help burn calories and increase muscle, strength, and flexibility. Stretching and lengthening muscles will help you feel more relaxed and help prevent muscle soreness. Stretching before bed will help relax your body and prepare you for sleep.

When you're conscious of how you feel and what causes you stress, steps can be taken to avoid stress and help your get through the day. When you know what to do to help you relax, take steps when you first experience the signs of stress. Increased heart rate, sweating, overheating, feeling flush, clenching teeth, frowning, and tense muscles are all signs of stress.

When these things start to happen, take a few minutes to pause and take 10 deep cleansing breaths, breathing in through your nose and out through your mouth. Concentrate on relaxing your body and slowing down your heart rate. This is such an incredible stress reliever that it may make you feel lightheaded.

When you're getting your blood pressure taken, deep breathing will bring down your blood pressure. If you're rushing to the doctor's office and your blood pressure reading is high, ask the nurse to let you retake it after taking 10 deep breaths. You'll be surprised how much this will bring down your blood pressure. Don't just do this when you get your blood pressure taken. Do it all the time to keep your blood pressure and heart rate down.

Stress causes many reactions in your body when you react to it negatively: your heart rate goes up, your blood pressure goes up, your muscles get tight, and your neck and jaw start to get tight. This can lead to problems with your back, neck, muscle spasms, headaches, temporomandibular joint dysfunction (TMJ), and grinding of the teeth, just to name a few.

Long-term stress or reacting in these ways to stress will cause elevated cortisol levels, weight gain, chronic back and neck pain, and problems with your teeth. When this pattern is repeated over a long period, more serious health problems can occur, such as high blood pressure, high cholesterol, heart disease, and type 2 diabetes. Chronic stress has even been linked to cancer. These are excellent reasons to learn to control your stress.

Knowing your personal triggers for stress can help you greatly reduce the negative effects of stress. Everyone reacts to stress in a different way and to different degrees, which makes this something you must learn about yourself. For some people, an event can be extremely stressful, while for others the same event appears as a minor obstacle. If you've been saving money all year to pay your taxes, April 15 will not be a stressful date. You have prepared to pay your yearly taxes or quarterly taxes if you own your own business, so you don't need to stress about taxes. If you haven't planned or prepared and you wait until April 14 to try to figure out your taxes and hope you have the money to pay them, this becomes very stressful.

I'm sure you'll find that the people who don't stress about taxes are the ones who prepare in advance and put money aside to pay taxes at the end of the year. These people aren't necessarily rich, but they have control because they planned. If you fail to plan, you plan to fail.

Planning also helps avoid unwanted weight gain and keep yourself physically fit. When you plan to be healthy and make the necessary life changes to keep yourself healthy, it's very easy to maintain your weight and avoid serious illness.

Many people believe that as they age, they'll become ill. This is not necessarily true if you're taking care of yourself by eating healthy and getting daily exercise. Avoiding unnecessary stress and dealing with stress in a positive way can help maintain a healthy weight and even increase your life span. Living longer and staying healthy are key to feeling great throughout your life. By making healthy living a priority and planning to live a long, healthy life, you'll be able to live a longer life.

Inactivity

Inactivity or being sedentary is one big reason people gain weight, but it's also the easiest to change. If you aren't getting some form of exercise every day, you're inactive and need to get up and start moving. Whether you need to lose weight, improve your health, or are maintaining a healthy lifestyle, exercise plays a very important role. A body in motion stays in motion. When you keep your body moving, the joints and muscles get lubricated and muscles become strong, which supports your skeletal system. Balance and flexibility are both very important, and exercise can help improve both. Joint pain is also very common in those who are overweight due to stress put on all the joints in the body to carry the excess weight.

Pain

One of the common mistakes is to do nothing about pain. The pain is your body under stress telling you something is out of balance. If you're overweight and have persistent joint pain, knee pain, back pain, or foot pain, losing weight can help you avoid surgery by taking the extra stress off your joints and spine.

Lower back pain is very common and can be caused by weak muscles, poor posture, and muscular strain, which can be improved with daily exercise. The more muscle you have, the better your body will be at holding itself up in a good posture, which takes the stress off the back.

Exercise is good for your weight-loss goals because when you exercise, you burn more calories, and you generally can eat more food and still lose weight. When you run for 30 minutes, you can burn from 200 to 500 calories. My actual number of calories burned from 60 minutes on my spinning bike is 500 to 575 calories. When I use the elliptical trainer at the gym, I burn 420 to 500 calories in an hour. Men will burn more calories in an hour because they have more muscle mass, which enables them to burn more calories.

Reducing stress and inactivity is good for your overall health and will reduce the cortisol produced by stress. The best way to reduce stress and inactivity is to exercise. Daily exercise can help you lose weight, and exercise also causes the body to release endorphins, which are the "feel good" hormones. The release of endorphins when you run makes you feel so good it's been called a "runner's high." This is a very healthy way to reduce stress and lose unwanted pounds.

Instead of telling yourself that it's too hard to start exercising or eat healthy, make one healthy change and stick with it. By adding more healthy things to your life, everything will fall into place. Make a list of healthy foods including lean protein like chicken breast, fish, ground turkey breast, nitrate-free oven-roasted turkey, or roast your own turkey or chicken. Fruits and vegetables contain vitamins and nutrients like phytochemicals that can only be found in nature. Add additional vitamins and fiber that are in fruits and vegetables. Buy 100% whole grains like brown rice, quinoa, Ezekiel Bread, Ezekiel tortilla shells, oatmeal, and oat flour along with any other healthy grain. Be sure to add legumes and beans, which can be bought in a can or dried to be cooked at home. This gives you a perfect start to a healthy eating plan you can do for the rest of your life.

Chapter 4: Lose Weight Quick – The Best Way to Eat

The best way to prevent diseases like diabetes or heart disease is to eat a healthy diet and get regular exercise before you gain weight or get an illness. If parents teach their children to eat healthy and get regular exercise and set a good example by doing the same, they can avoid many illnesses and diseases. When you start life with good habits, they'll stick with you throughout your life. I don't know anyone who wants to be overweight or unhealthy.

By looking at food as fuel for your body, it takes away the temptation to eat unhealthy junk and fast foods. When you exercise, you know that your body needs fuel to get through your routine, whether it's weightlifting, running, team sports, or dance classes. The fuel your body needs comes in the form of healthy carbohydrates, lean proteins, and a small amount of healthy fat. This is what your body needs to run efficiently. If you don't give your body the nutrients it needs, problems will arise.

Having a healthy eating plan like the one I recommend will help you lose weight and stop craving sugar, junk, and fast foods because your body will be satisfied and feel full. People who go on fad diets and lose weight are losing water weight in the beginning and then burning muscle for energy. The less muscle mass you have, the slower your metabolism will be. Therefore, athletes consume a lot of calories, and with their muscle mass, their bodies burn the calories efficiently.

Don't look at the diet of someone like a professional athlete and think you can have a cheat day like theirs. It takes a lot of calories and hard training to build that type of muscle. Actors and famous people have personal chefs, personal trainers, and assistants that help keep them in the shape they're in. They make it seem easy, but they also have plastic surgery and other treatments to keep them looking young and fit. They don't have special genes or a magic potion. They don't use a certain face cream or drink aloe vera juice or Gatorade and look the way they do. They must always look their best in their profession, and the industry uses everything available to achieve that image.

There's nothing wrong with that fact unless they tell the public that they look timeless or ageless due to using certain products. They undergo any type of procedure and plastic surgery to make themselves look great all the time. They may claim they never went under the knife, but if you see a show they were on years ago and they don't have the same nose, face, cheekbones, or body they previously had, they may have had plastic surgery. This doesn't mean they're healthy because they look better than ever. If a person wants plastic surgery, that is their choice, but don't say it's natural for people to not age. Eating healthy is your best defense against the signs of aging.

Weight loss
When celebrities say they work hard to get their bodies in shape for a role, it may be true, or it may be plastic surgery. When a

woman loses weight, excess fat in the breast tissue goes down, making the breast size a bit smaller. Women who lift weights a lot may notice they lose breast size due to the initial reduction of fat, but the body becomes firmer and stronger. Also, their bottoms will initially get smaller along with the rest of the body as they become sculpted and toned. When a celebrity loses weight and has the same big round bottom and big bust, it is plastic surgery.

There is no such thing as spot reducing. When you lose weight, it comes off all over. Some people, especially women, may have problem areas that take longer to lose fat from, but weight loss is typically throughout the body. You can't compare yourself to the fake women you see on television or in magazines.

Men are also joining in on plastic surgery with Botox to get rid of wrinkles (it paralyzes the muscles in the face), facelifts, hair restoration, and whatever means available to keep themselves looking young. Remember, a pleasant appearance does not always indicate good health. Eating healthy and exercising achieves both goals of looking our best while increasing our overall healthy lifestyle.

The starting point of any change in habit is to start immediately by taking some form of action toward achieving your goal. The goal should be to become a healthy, active person and sustain your health throughout your life. Looking great is just a perk of exercise and healthy eating. One of the gyms in the 1990s had a shirt for sale to advertise their gym that said "Look Better Naked." Anyone can make themselves look good in clothes, spanx, blousy tops, or tight clothes that hold in the fat.

I had a friend who said you should have a lot of mirrors in your house so you can always be checking yourself to make sure you look good. That's a really good idea. Many people avoid mirrors, especially full-length mirrors that show their bodies. You want to be proud of your body and feel good about yourself. Even if you aren't exactly where you want to be, check in with yourself and ask what you can do to change the things you need to. Don't accept less than a healthy body and a long, healthy life.

Scales are necessary to help avoid weight gain and provide feedback that is necessary for your health. Keeping track of your weight and how you look will provide the motivation needed to keep you on the right track. The only reason to avoid the mirror or the scale is if you already know you need to lose weight and don't want to face the fact. It's better to know where you are and what's working than to avoid the facts. Whether you need to lose weight or just want to improve your muscle or appearance, checking in a mirror and on a scale will help.

Stretch pants, especially stretch jeans, only make people think they're not gaining weight because they can still fit into their pants. Save the skinny jeans and buy clothes that fit well without room to grow wider. Stretchy clothes mask the fact that you're gaining unwanted weight and need to cut out the foods or junk foods that are causing you to gain weight. When you know where you should be and want to be with your weight, stay there. Don't let those pounds creep up on you; it's easier to lose a few pounds than 40, 50, or 100 pounds. This is a slippery slope that you don't want to go down. Cut down when you start to gain weight, and get back on track with your healthy eating and exercise.

Gaining weight can happen over a month or over the years, but either way, it's not good for your health. I have found that many people expect to gain weight and continue to gain weight as they age. There is no reason to gain weight as you age. Staying active and eating healthy will keep you from gaining weight. It has been proven that people of any age can gain muscle by doing weight-bearing exercises like lifting weights. The more muscle you have, the more calories you'll burn. Playing sports like tennis and basketball are also ways to stay in shape and keep the pounds off.

Making changes in your life is easier than you may think, and all it takes is a little planning. By planning your meals, you can easily stick to my healthy eating plan and not worry about counting calories, cutting out carbs, or cutting out meals. You will never go hungry or starve yourself to lose weight. The pounds will easily come off when you give your body the fuel it needs.

Body weight

Weighing yourself once a week will keep you on track. The number on the scale will vary from one person to the other depending on the amount of muscle they have, their gender, and activity level. A bodybuilder who lifts heavy weights will weigh more than someone else who's the same height because muscle weighs more than fat. Many scales measure your weight and percentage of body fat. This is a good way to track your progress whether you're trying to lose weight or just need to maintain your weight.

It's very difficult to use clothing as a gauge due to stretchy fabrics and variations in sizes. If you have old jeans that aren't stretch denim, they can also be a handy tool to let you know if you're gaining weight. I had clients tell me that they didn't know they were fat or gaining weight even though they went from a size two to a size 10. One woman told me her face never got fat, so she didn't realize she was 200 pounds overweight. People are different in size, shape, and weight for many reasons, and they may not be able to grasp the fact that they've gained a lot of weight and need to lose weight. Use the scale at least once a week to check your weight and make sure you're staying at a healthy weight.

Heart rate monitors are popular and useful when you work out. I use a heart rate monitor by Polar. The important thing is that the watch gives your heart rate, the number of calories burned, and the percent of fat burned during your workout. This is an effective motivational tool. I have been using the Polar heart rate monitor since 1994 when I started running. It lets you challenge yourself and keeps track of how many calories you burn during a workout. It also lets you know your fat-burning range. I write my numbers down on my diet and exercise log every day. The process of manually transcribing the data is a method of being tactilely engaged and is another way to stay motivated and track progress. I also write my weight and body fat down one or two times a week. I can look back at the years of using Tracy's Healthy Eating Plan and my exercise and see that I've maintained a healthy body weight over the years just by eating healthy foods and exercising.

Why start eating healthy now? Because every day that you procrastinate is another day of overeating, which leads to weight gain. Be proactive by taking steps to reduce the amount of saturated fat, junk foods, and sugary snacks. It only takes a few changes to start to make a big difference. Cut out the cream, sugar, and flavorings in your coffee, and stop eating donuts, cakes, and pastries. This reduces calories, and you won't miss the unhealthy foods if you replace them with tasty foods like plain yogurt and fresh fruit, low-fat cottage cheese, rice cakes, and veggie chips. There are so many healthy snacks that can replace all the junk foods.

Making healthy versions of things that you like to eat will make it easy to change your eating habits. Eat ground turkey breast or a veggie patty instead of ground beef. Grill or bake your chicken instead of frying it. Eat flourless bread like Ezekiel Bread or Alvarado Street. Making small changes will greatly reduce the number of calories in your meals and the amount of saturated fat. Changes to your body and attitude will show very quickly. You'll feel better and look better, making you wonder why you haven't been eating healthy all your life.

There are many ways to lose weight, and some work better than others, but one thing is true no matter what diet you try: the right way to lose weight is to eat healthy foods and exercise. When you burn more calories than you consume, you will lose weight. This does not mean starving yourself or eating a very low-calorie diet. When you eat whole foods in their natural state without sauces, sugar, and artificial ingredients, your body will use the calories from the food for vital functions and energy. A calorie is a measurement of energy. Fruits and vegetables are low in calories and full of fiber and vitamins and minerals that are vital for good health.

Reading labels or looking up nutritional values on the computer before you go to the store will help you make the best choices for your family. Don't let advertisers sway your decision-making process. Choosing quality foods that have no added sugars, preservatives, artificial colors, or ingredients that you can't pronounce. Be smart about what you buy. You are what you eat, so eat the best foods in their natural state, eat a lot of organic fruits and vegetables, whole grains, and only lean protein. This makes it easy to avoid chemicals, preservatives, and herbicides that are put on conventional produce, which are harmful to your health and have been proven to cause cancer. Many of these have been outlawed in the U. S., but produce imported from other counties may have these harmful chemicals, which is why buying organic, fresh, and local produce is best.

Cutting hidden calories
A calorie is a measurement of energy used by your body to keep its systems running. If you don't eat enough calories, your body can't run efficiently. If you eat more calories than your body

requires to function, you'll gain weight. If the calories you consume are made up of mostly fast foods and junk foods, you will not only gain weight but you will also gain fat and set yourself up for future problems such as obesity, type 2 diabetes, high blood sugar, high cholesterol, high blood pressure, heart disease, and even cancer. Eating junk foods and fast foods that are high in fat, sodium, sugar, preservatives, artificial ingredients and low in nutrients can cause many types of problems. Your body was created to run on carbohydrates, protein, and fat. When you eat complex carbohydrates such as 100% whole grain breads and cereals, brown rice, whole grain pastas and vegetables, your body has the proper fuel to operate efficiently.

Excessive use of condiments or dressings adds a lot of extra calories and unhealthy fat to otherwise healthy meals. Extra calories are also added when you add fatty sugary toppings like whipped cream, flavorings, caramel, cream, or sugar to coffee or tea drinks. Plain coffee has 2.4 calories per cup, but when you add a serving of whipped cream, this adds 82 calories, eight grams of fat, and five grams of saturated fat per 22 grams of whipped cream.

If you don't add whipped cream, you're cutting almost 100 calories and eight grams of fat from one drink. If you skip the crust of a pie and the whipped cream, especially if it's a pumpkin pie, you'll be eating the pumpkin and not the fatty crust and whipped cream, which reduces the calories. To make an even healthier version of pumpkin pie, make your own with stevia and eliminate the sugar and the extra calories. Making small changes can dramatically reduce your overall caloric intake. If you want to lose weight, you need to burn or use more calories than you consume.

The body needs a certain number of calories just to stay alive. If your body doesn't get the calories it needs to stay alive, it will slow down the metabolism and start storing fat. If you consistently eat fewer calories than the body needs, the body thinks it's starving and stores fat to be used slowly as the metabolism slows down and uses fewer calories. This is not a state you want to be in because the body will start breaking down muscles to use for energy. When you have less muscle, your metabolism slows down.

People who try to lose weight by fasting or restricting calories to a very low level will lose weight at first, but this will be in the form of water weight. If the lack of calories continues, the body will start to use muscle as fuel. Again, this will show weight loss on the scale because muscle weighs more than fat. This is not the way to lose weight. Sacrificing muscle to lose weight by eating a diet very low in calories will create a lot of problems for you, especially if you're constantly dieting and losing weight and then putting the weight back on. This type of yoyo dieting will slow your metabolism and cause your body to stay at a set number of pounds in anticipation of the next fasting or low-calorie diet.

Portion control

Portion size is very important, and it makes it very easy to cut calories by using a nine-inch plate and using half of the plate for steamed veggies and salad, one quarter of the plate for starchy carbohydrates like brown rice or sweet potatoes, and the other quarter for lean protein. The rule of thumb is lean protein the size of a deck of cards or the size of your palm, starchy carbohydrates the size of your fist (without butter or oil), and healthy oil the size of the end of your thumb from knuckle to tip. This makes portion control simple and easy for everyone.

Remember, if you're working out hard every day or training for a race or play sports regularly, you can increase your intake of protein and carbohydrates. If you start gaining fat instead of muscle, you need to cut back. If you're losing weight but not gaining muscle, you need to increase your protein or work out harder.

Your body will crave what it needs. Let your body tell you what it needs to run smoothly. When you feel hungry, a meal with lean protein and healthy complex carbohydrates will make you feel satisfied. If your energy level is low, eat half a yam, and a small bowl of brown rice or Ezekiel Sesame Bread made by Food for Life. Any of their breads are ideal for a quick pick-up without a crash later because they are flourless and have protein and fiber with 100% whole grains and legumes, organic wheat, barley, soybeans, and lentils (all sprouted). Ezekiel Bread has no flour and contains all nine essential amino acids. If you have any gluten sensitivities, stick with yams, squash, quinoa, and gluten-free grains.

The best way to lose weight and keep it off is to eat foods that are high in nutrients and low in calories. Fruits and vegetables are packed with vitamins and fiber, along with phytochemicals that are only found in nature. Fruits and vegetables are low in calories and have vital nutrients. Focus on a variety of colors on your plate to ensure you're getting all the nutrients your body needs to function.

It's very easy to lose weight when you cut out all the junk foods in your diet. Start by cleaning out your pantry and refrigerator and eliminating anything that has artificial ingredients, colors, and preservatives. Read the label to look for artificial ingredients, trans fats, high-fructose corn syrup, MSG, and other chemicals that are harmful to the body and to your efforts to lose weight. Make a clean sweep of processed foods and junk foods.

Do whatever you need to do to get rid of them. Out of sight, out of mind. Don't give in to temptations when you're home or when you go to the store. These things don't benefit your body and keep you from losing weight. The chemicals in junk foods aren't good for the body. Every time you think about eating anything, ask yourself if it's good for your body.

Cheat days and trigger foods

Everyone wants to have cheat days when they're on a diet, which is one of the reasons diets don't work. Cheat days imply that you can eat whatever you want all day long. This can sabotage your diet and weight loss as well as reinforce a bad habit. The reason you're trying to lose weight is because you gained weight eating the way you eat and the foods you eat. If you go back to those foods every week, you might as well not try to change your bad eating habits. Eating healthy all the time will help you stay slim and healthy without worrying about whether you're going to gain weight or not.

Many professional athletes, Olympians, or those who have a rigorous training schedule have a lot of muscle, which enables them to burn more calories. This is not something that normal people can do weekly without gaining weight or risking health issues. Many professional athletes have trainers, chefs, and assistants that help them stay in top shape. Don't compare yourself to professional athletes or aspire to look just like them. Either it will become a dangerous obsession or you'll fail miserably. Knowing that eating healthy and exercising will get you to where you need to be will keep you grounded.

Cheat days have more serious downfalls, and one of them is using food as a reward for good behavior. Never use food as a reward for anything. It is crucial for you and your children to know food is not a reward. Food is something you give your body so that you can function at an optimal level and stay healthy. Children who have been given desserts and sugary snacks for good behavior will end up doing the same thing when they get older. They'll go straight for sugary snacks when something goes well and unhealthy foods during times of low mood to make themselves feel better. Before you know it, they have a weight problem and an unhealthy attachment to food. This can lead to eating disorders like binge eating and purging. *Do not use food as a REWARD.* This will give you an unhealthy attachment to food. A reward should be to go to the park, play a game, or visit a friend, not junk food like pastries, cake, pie, or other sugary, fatty junk foods.

The cheat day is something that can also cause problems because many people have foods that trigger them to eat more. Trigger foods are foods that make you lose control when you eat them. Sugary, fatty, and salty snacks can be trigger foods. When you eat junk foods out of a large bag, it's hard to gauge how much you're eating, and before you know it, the entire bag is gone. These snacks aren't satisfying because they contain no fiber, little to no nutrients, and are high in sodium, artificial ingredients, artificial color, preservatives, and sugar. Potato chips, Cheetos, Doritos, and any other junk food that falls into this category should be eliminated from your diet, especially if they contain fake yellow or orange powdered cheese and spices. They are harmful to the body and cause you to want to eat more of them. They can be very addictive.

Snack companies are in business to make money, not to provide a healthy meal or snack. They don't want you to be able to resist eating the whole bag. The only thing worse than eating potato chips, Doritos, and other junk chips is putting dip or salad dressing on them. Now your appetite is stimulated by salt, sugar, and fat along with artificial flavoring and coloring, and many contain HFCS, which keeps your body from producing the hormone Leptin, which tells your body to stop eating because you're full. These are horrible for adults and even more harmful to children.

Some people say when they eat certain foods like chips or cake, they want to eat more. The sugar and salt in these items can cause cravings because you acquire a taste for them. When you eat a lot of salt, it makes everything without salt taste bland, which will make you crave more salty foods. The same thing happens when you eat sugar. Foods with added sugars like cake, candy, and pastries make you crave more sugar. They cause a spike in your blood sugar, and then it drops, leaving you craving more sugar.

Gillian Michaels, the trainer from *The Biggest Loser*, wrote a book after discovering she had a problem with her thyroid, and she claims that this fake yellow-orange powder damages the thyroid. This is your master hormone producer that controls a lot of functions in the body. Why would you want to put artificial ingredients into your body?

Cheat days are like deciding to stop smoking cigarettes three days a week and smoking the other four days. You'll never kick the habit that way. This reinforces the bad behavior because you're rewarding yourself with the very thing you're trying to stop doing. Be clear in your mind that you must stop smoking or chewing tobacco because it is unhealthy and you are *never* going to use tobacco again. This is how you quit a bad habit. Replace the bad habit with something good for you like exercise. Stop smoking or chewing tobacco and never look back. Look forward to a healthy, happy new life without these bad habits.

When you want to change a bad habit, whether it's to stop smoking, drinking, or overeating, it's important to link a positive feeling to the habit you want to create and a negative image of the one you want to quit. Having a cheat day means you're looking forward to doing something you shouldn't do. Visualize yourself looking good in a bathing suit to help you lose weight. Visualize yourself with beautiful white teeth and beautiful skin when you stop smoking. Whatever you attach a positive image and feeling to will help you achieve your goal. Visualize and act as if you already have what you want to make your reality.

Planning cheat days keeps you hooked on eating things that you're trying to avoid, so why not just eliminate foods that are unhealthy? Substitute fruit for French fries, brown rice for white rice, and baked or broiled chicken instead of fried chicken. By making small substitutions in your daily meals, the total calorie count of the meal goes down as well as your weekly calorie count. This is how you can lose weight and still eat some of the things you like—or at least a healthier version of the things you like to eat.

The key is planning and knowing in advance so you can make smart food choices. Once you get in the habit of doing this, it will be simple to eat healthy regardless of where you are.

Making positive changes to your meal plan can result in fast changes to your weight and energy level. When you eat whole foods and make healthy food choices, your body has the energy it needs to function and keep you going all day long. When you step on the scale or try on those pants that were too tight, it will be obvious that these changes are working for you.

Chapter 5: Daily Meals

Cutting calories out of your daily meals may seem hard to do, but it's quite simple. Making healthy food choices will enable you to cut calories and not notice the difference because you'll be replacing high-calorie foods with low-calorie foods that are good for you. The fiber in fruits, vegetables, and 100% whole grains keeps you feeling full longer and contains fewer calories than processed and fast foods.

There are many ways to cut calories and make a meal taste good and be good for you. When you leave out fatty meats and pork products such as bacon, sausage, and fatty beef, your meals will have less fat and fewer calories. Turkey or chicken breast can be used in many recipes that have beef in them. Ground turkey breast is 99% fat-free, and regular ground turkey meat with light and dark meat is better than beef or pork. Eat vegetarian meals to cut down the calories. Just replacing one meal a day with vegetables, beans, legumes, and brown rice will significantly reduce your overall calorie intake.

It's very easy to make inexpensive meat-free meals. Chile beans, lima beans, navy beans, lentils, split peas, and a variety of vegetables can all be made into delicious soup without any meat.

You may have heard of bone broth, which is what many celebrities are talking about. It is just using bones to make soup, which people have done for hundreds of years. The bones from chicken or beef cooked in a slow cooker or on the stovetop on low make a tasty broth. Put it in the refrigerator, and the saturated fat gets hard and becomes a layer on top of the broth. Scoop the fat off and use the broth. The fat can also be skimmed off the top while cooking, which looks like oil sitting on top of the broth. Fresh or frozen vegetables can be added to the broth to give it texture, fiber, and vitamins.

When it comes to changing your eating habits, find healthy versions of things you like to eat. You can make foods that are healthy versions of the foods you're leaving out of your diet. Make a turkey or veggie burger on Ezekiel toast or bread with mustard, lettuce, tomato, and agave ketchup. This is a very healthy way to have your burger. Instead of French fries, have fruit, or baked or microwaved potatoes. Cut them like home or French fries, put them on a cookie sheet or tin foil lightly sprayed with cooking spray, and broil them in the oven until golden brown. Serve alongside your healthy burger. Use a small amount of agave ketchup or buy unsweetened ketchup and sweeten it with a little stevia leaf. If you're diabetic and can't have ketchup, the unsweetened ketchup with stevia leaf powder mixed in is an option for you. Instead of eating Yukon Gold potatoes, eat Japanese or garnet sweet potatoes. These can be cut and put on a baking sheet and cooked just like Yukon Gold potatoes. Other options for diabetics are non-starchy vegetables or coleslaw made without mayo or sugar.

Oily fish such as salmon, tuna, sardines, mackerel, and trout are full of omega-3 fatty acids. These fish should be a staple in your diet. I could eat salmon every day and be happy. If you like bagels with lox and cream cheese, skip the cream cheese or put a very light smear of it on the bagel and buy a whole-grain bagel instead of one made from white flour. Remember, white flour and water make paste. I would suggest skipping the cream cheese or at least choosing a light cream cheese and use sparingly, and make the bagel an Ezekiel Bagel. Just make a few little changes, and you're eating healthier already.

A fried chicken breast with skin has 260 calories, 9.43 grams of carbohydrates, 13.29 grams of fat, and 943 grams of protein. A skinless grilled breast that is four ounces has 110 calories, three grams of fat, one gram of saturated fat, 23 grams of protein, and zero carbohydrates. The carbohydrates of the fried chicken come from the flour that the chicken is rolled into before frying. By removing the skin from chicken and baking or broiling the chicken, you eliminate not just calories but unnecessary and unhealthy fat from your meal. Anytime you make a meal, remove the fatty skin, bake, broil, or barbeque, and leave the breading off.

Chicken, fish, or ground turkey can be broiled, baked, grilled, or prepared on a stovetop. I also like to use my stovetop to prepare many of the meals I serve. It's quick and easy to prepare meals on the stovetop in a skillet, fry, or wok pan without any butter or oil. If you do use oil, make sure its' a high-quality oil, and use it sparingly. This will count in your overall calorie count and the amount of fat you eat for the day. Use a non-stick pan or spray a little olive oil cooking spray, or wipe the pan with a little olive oil to prevent sticking. Remember the amount of oil you should eat in a day is the size of the end of your thumb, which is a very small amount. It doesn't take much to keep the food from sticking and to keep your calorie count down.

When eating at a restaurant, order your food with no breading, butter, oil, seasoning, dressings, or sauces. Restaurants are in business to make money, and whatever they can put on your food to make it taste good, they will use. Food is cooked with oil that is cheap, not healthy, and the amount of sodium is very high. Most dressings, sauces, and seasonings at restaurants, and some store-bought, have artificial ingredients and flavor enhancers like monosodium glutamate (MSG). Many people are sensitive to MSG and can experience racing heart, headaches, and nausea. It has been deemed safe to put in food, but why take the risk? These flavor enhancers also cause people to eat more than they normally do.

HFCS is used for sweetener and is used in many processed foods. HFCS stops the body from producing leptin, the hormone that makes you feel full, which leads to overeating. Always avoid HFCS, which is used by many restaurants and is in processed and fast foods. If you feel a little seasoning is needed, add a light dusting of salt and pepper if you don't have any heart issues or other medical restrictions. Put it on when you get your food so you can control the amount, and only use a pinch. Most foods made at a restaurant are cooked with a lot of oil that's not high in quality. Ordering meals without oil cuts a lot of calories and fat from your meals.

Preparing your own food is the best way to make sure you're getting all the fresh, healthy ingredients without artificial colors and flavorings. Choose low-sodium foods, and base your meals around fresh or frozen fruits and vegetables, and buy organic, at least the "dirty dozen" that contain the highest number of pesticides and herbicides. These are strawberries, spinach, kale, collard and mustard greens, nectarines, apples, grapes, bell and hot peppers, cherries, peaches, pears, celery, and tomatoes, which should always be organically grown. Fruits with a hard outer shell, like melons, can be conventionally grown instead of organically grown if you're trying to save money. Look at some of the things that you spend money on like magazines, tobacco, alcohol, expensive coffees, eating out, and fast food and determine how much money you spend on unnecessary items. Put that money toward buying organic produce.

When it comes to organic products, read the label and make wise decisions. Do you need to buy organic candy or cookies? The best thing to do is to avoid candy and cookies altogether. Snack on fresh fruit and vegetables, and eat healthy meals, which will eliminate cravings for salty and sweet snacks. Make the largest part of your meal vegetables that are non-starchy, like broccoli, cauliflower, cabbage, and carrots, and eat as many of them as you want. Make a healthy salad and add a variety of vegetables to add a lot of nutrients. Romaine lettuce, spinach, red cabbage, broccoli, cauliflower, cucumber, garbanzo beans, kidney beans, artichokes, and hearts of palm packed in water, not oil, make a healthy meal that you can enjoy anytime.

Vegetables
Vegetables like broccoli, cauliflower, carrots, celery, mushrooms, bell peppers, and radishes are all good to eat raw or use in a salad to add extra crunch. Crunchy vegetables make a healthy snack that you can take with you in a plastic bag or container. Vegetables are packed with vitamins and fiber that are necessary for good health and aid in digestion. Cruciferous vegetables like broccoli, cauliflower, cabbage, Brussels sprouts, and leafy greens fight cancer. Be sure to add at least one of these vegetables every day or use them in a stir fry—or what I love to make, an "unfry," because I never fry anything. By using water and Bragg's Amino Acids, I can eliminate the oil and cut down on calories and fat. Add some cooked shrimp, fermented tofu, or cooked chicken breast for a tasty, satisfying meal. Brown rice and quinoa are other additions to

this dish and add more fiber and nutrients, making a filling meal.

Making coleslaw is easy, especially if you buy the bag of pre-chopped cabbage or coleslaw. Add red wine, apple cider, or balsamic vinegar, onion salt or powder, and garlic powder or fresh garlic. This gives it a flavor with cancer-fighting nutrients while being extremely low in calories. This is good in the summer or even in the winter to keep in your refrigerator as a side dish or snack. There is an olive oil or low-fat mayonnaise which you can use sparingly, but it adds fat and calories to the coleslaw, which can be taken to picnics or shared with others.

Healthy snacks like fruit or berries with organic plain Greek yogurt and a little stevia leaf can be enjoyed anytime. Fruit is also good with low-fat, organic cottage cheese. I like to cut up an apple and add a spoon of cottage cheese. Eating protein with your fruit helps keep your blood sugar from spiking. Eliminating sugar and salty snacks is a good way to keep you from food cravings, and eating protein with your meals and snacks will help you build muscle and keep you feeling full longer. Eating lean protein and healthy carbohydrates will be a benefit to your mental capacity and your weight loss goals.

Fruits

Fruits, vegetables, and 100% whole grains contain the vitamins, minerals, and fiber necessary to stay healthy. Fruits are considered a simple carbohydrate because of their naturally occurring sugar. Fruits contain phytochemicals, as do vegetables that are vital to health and can only be found in nature. You cannot take a vitamin to replace a whole food.

Diabetics have limits of around 200 grams of carbohydrates per day. Fruits may need to be limited due to the 15 grams of carbohydrates they contain. The blood glucose index (GI) is a ranking of carbohydrates in foods according to how they affect blood sugar levels. Glycemic carbohydrates with a low GI value (55 or less) are more slowly digested, absorbed, and metabolized and cause a lower and slower rise in the blood glucose index.

Some fruits are higher on the glycemic index, which rates the amount of sugar in each type of fruit and vegetable. Bananas and watermelon are high in sugar, so they're high on the glycemic index. Many fruits are low in carbohydrates, such as cantaloupe, avocados, honeydew, and peaches. Strawberries and other berries are loaded with nutrients and are low in carbohydrates. Complex carbohydrates that help you lose weight are the ones high in fiber like barley, whole-wheat or whole-grain pasta, acorn squash, legumes, whole-wheat bread or 100% whole-grain breads, black beans, oatmeal, and quinoa, which is also high in protein.

Dairy

Milk has naturally occurring sugar, which is called lactose. The protein in milk slows down the absorption of the lactose. The protein and calcium in milk helps grow strong bones, muscle, teeth, and hair. It also contains vitamin D, vitamin A, and lactic acid, which help to make skin look younger and softer.

Choosing the proper dairy product is important. When it comes to reducing calories, nonfat milk has 80 calories and 0.5% fat. Low-fat milk has 100 calories and is 1-1.5% fat. Full-fat milk has 150 calories and five grams of fat.

Eating fewer calories will help to lose weight, and eating less fat can help reduce the risk of cardiovascular disease. When you're trying to lose weight, consuming fewer calories will help, so choose nonfat for the least number of calories. Low-fat comes in 2% or 1% fat, which is the next lowest in the number of calories. Full-fat will have the highest amount of fat and calories.

There are arguments for and against full-fat dairy. The choice is up to you, and in the end, if you're trying to consume fewer calories per day to lose weight, you may be better off using the nonfat or low-fat version of dairy products during your weight loss. Consuming dairy products is far more healthy than choosing soft drinks like sodas. All soda, whether it's sugar-free or has sugar, is unnecessary and provides no health benefits. Sugar causes cavities, and artificial sugar is so sweet it can lead to being unsatisfied with the natural sweetness of fruit and things that are good for you.

Nondairy choices are almond milk, oat milk, or soy milk, which are enhanced with nutrients. For infants, breast milk is the best, and young children do need to drink milk unless they are eating foods that are high in calcium and protein to give them healthy bones and teeth. Spinach and cabbage are a good source of calcium and protein. Children who don't get enough calcium and protein have small or malformed teeth and weak bones. Drinking milk and eating vegetables makes it easy to get the necessary calcium to grow strong and healthy.

Organic dairy doesn't have the added hormones that are given to regular cows. I use organic nonfat milk or almond milk on cereal, nonfat or low-fat Greek yogurt, and low-fat cottage cheese in some of the meals I prepare. All milk has 12 grams of naturally occurring sugar, known as lactose. Whole milk has 145 calories and eight grams of fat. Choose fewer calories when trying to lose weight. People who are concerned with high performance and don't need to lose weight may choose to use whole milk.

Nuts

Nuts are good for you but have a lot of calories, fat, and contain some sugar. Nuts contain sucrose, which is naturally occurring sugar in sugar cane. Nuts contain two to six grams of sucrose, depending on the type of nut, per 100 grams. If the nuts are party nuts or coated nuts, they contain added sugar and a lot more calories. Raw nuts that have no added sugar are the best choice. Limit your nuts to eight almonds or walnuts, and skip the nuts that contain the most amount of fat. A serving of 10-12 macadamia nuts has two grams of protein and 21 grams of fat, and 18-20 pecan halves have three grams of protein and 20 grams of fat. Using nuts as a topping or garnish by sprinkling some slivered almonds on top of your oatmeal or using 1/4 or 1/3 cup (instead of 1/2 cup) of nuts in your favorite bread recipe will cut down on the total calories.

Nut butter
Add a little fat and protein to your rice cake or Ezekiel Bread, using nut butter sparingly. Nut butter has more calories, but when used sparingly, it can help reduce cravings and keep you feeling full. Brown rice cakes with a smear of almond or Better'n Peanut Butter is a wonderful snack that is low in sodium and sugar compared to peanut butter, and it's also lower in fat. This healthy fat can help you feel full longer than a rice cake alone. One organic slightly salted brown rice cake has about 60 calories.

Two tablespoons of peanut butter or almond butter is a lot of calories and fat. It only takes a small amount of nut butter to give you the flavor you crave. Two tablespoons of almond butter by Whole Foods 365 brand has 190 calories: 150 calories from fat, 12 grams of total fat, 1.5 saturated fat, four grams of polyunsaturated fat, 10 grams of monounsaturated fat, seven grams of carbohydrates, two grams of sugar, and seven grams of protein. Better'n Peanut Butter (a lower fat and calorie peanut butter) has 100 calories per two tablespoons, 20 calories from fat, two grams of total fat, zero saturated fat, zero trans-fat, one gram of polyunsaturated fat, one gram of monounsaturated fat, 12 grams of carbohydrates, two grams of fiber, and four grams of protein. This is just an example of nutritional facts. Amounts vary with different brands. Nuts and olive oil have healthy monounsaturated fats, but many mainstream brands add palm oil and a lot of sugar to their peanut butter. Read the labels and check the ingredients to find the best products.

Oil

Oils have almost two times the calories of carbohydrates. When you bake, use applesauce instead of oil, which cuts down on calories and fat. If you must use oil, do so sparingly and choose a high-quality oil like extra virgin olive or canola oil, which are low in saturated fat. Flax seed oil, grape seed oil, and avocado oil are also good oils to use.

Yogurt

Yogurt is another product that varies from brand to brand. Read the labels and buy Greek yogurt if you need more protein. Buy plain yogurt and sweeten it with stevia leaf, and put fresh berries on top instead of buying flavored yogurt, which has added sugar and may contain artificial ingredients. This can make a big difference in the amount of sugar and the quality of the yogurt you're eating. It's less expensive and has fewer calories.

Sauces, gravies, butter, and condiments

Sauces, gravies, butter, and condiments are high in sugar, fat, artificial ingredients, and preservatives in many cases. Sauces and ketchup should be used sparingly or not at all, and you should always buy organic.

Many mayonnaise brands are high in fat, and sauces like

barbeque sauce are high in sugar, HFCS, and may have MSG. The organic brands usually do not have these ingredients, but be sure to check the label. It's very easy to make your own barbeque sauce and use stevia or xylitol instead of sugar. If you want to put a little on your chicken, wait until it's almost done and add a little during the last few minutes of cooking.

Two easy sauce recipes

Easy barbeque sauce can be made with 2 ½ ounces of tomato paste, 1/2 cup cider vinegar, 1/3 cup of xylitol, two tablespoons of Worcestershire sauce, one tablespoon of hickory smoke, two teaspoons of paprika or smoked paprika, one teaspoon of garlic powder, and 1/2 teaspoon of onion powder.

Low-fat hollandaise sauce can be made with one cup low-fat, plain, or nonfat yogurt, two teaspoons of lemon, three egg yolks or one egg yolk and two egg whites, or you can use liquid egg whites. Beat the lemon and egg yolks with the yogurt and mix well. Cook in a saucepan or use a strainer/sieve over a saucepan of water and place bowl in the sieve. Simmer, stirring frequently until sauce has thickened, which is 12-14 minutes. Remove from heat and stir in 1/4 teaspoon of Celtic or Himalayan salt, 1/2 teaspoon of Dijon mustard, and 1/2 turn from a pepper grinder.

This is easy and cuts a lot of calories from eggs benedict. I have my recipe for Tracy's Eggs Benedict in my *Healthy Meals in Minutes* book. Use an Ezekiel English muffin or a slice of Ezekiel sesame bread, poach one or two eggs, and heat a slice or two of thick-sliced nitrate-free deli turkey breast, or use leftover turkey from one that you roasted. Put it on top of the toasted muffin or bread and put a poached egg on top.

It takes about two to three minutes on low boil to poach an egg. If you want to make this vegetarian, which is also lower in calories, skip the turkey and add a slice of tomato and some spinach. Cooked eggplant can also be used in place of turkey.

Grains

Grains should always be 100% whole grains to get the most nutrients. Brown rice is a better option than white rice because it contains more fiber. Quinoa is a grain with a different taste than rice and is high in protein. Quinoa makes a good grain to use instead of or along with brown rice. Some natural food stores will combine brown rice and quinoa in brown rice sushi, which gives it more protein and a bit of a nutty flavor. It tastes fabulous and it is good for you. This grain can be used as a side dish or main dish by adding vegetables and tofu or chicken.

Bread

There are many different types of bread, and each contains a variety of ingredients which makes reading the label very important. If the label of ingredients is a paragraph long and contains words you never heard of don't buy that bread. The label should say 100% whole grains.

Whole wheat is not the same as 100% whole grain. You can tell the difference by the texture of the bread which is light and spongy and there is a mixture of wheat and white flour which you will not find in 100% whole grain bread. The bread should not have any artificial ingredients or preservatives, no trans fats and no sugar. Some types of bread do have sugar or other types of sweeteners added to make it taste better.

My favorite bread is Ezekiel bread which is a flourless bread made with 100% whole grains and legumes and all natural ingredients no preservatives or artificial ingredients. Many stores carry this bread in the freezer section of the store. Alvarado Street is another bread that is flourless and made with all natural ingredients. Both brands are tasty and nutrient dense. The spongy, soft breads have white and wheat flour have a lot of artificial ingredients to make them soft and preservatives to give them a longer shelf life. There is also a very little fiber in white flour products compared to 100% whole grains.

Tortillas

All tortillas are not created equal, and it's important to look for the Ezekiel or Alvarado Street brands, which are high in fiber and have a pleasing flavor and texture. Instead of doughy white flour tortillas, you have more satisfying tortillas made with whole grains that contain fiber and help you feel and stay full longer than the white flour products. Some stores now have their own brands of whole-wheat tortillas, but they're not flourless, and they don't have the fiber and flavor of Ezekiel or Alvarado Street tortillas. I ordered Ezekiel tortillas online and didn't see the size of the box, which had 20 packages of tortillas inside. Luckily, I have a variety of meals I can make with tortillas, and I had room in the freezer for the rest.

Gluten-free

Gluten-free products are usually higher in calories and low in nutrients because they're highly processed. Try making your own bread and add flax meal, which is high in fiber. One tablespoon of ground flaxseed is about seven grams and contains two grams of polyunsaturated fatty acids (including omega-3), two grams of fiber, and 37 calories. Flaxseed is commonly used to improve digestive health and relieve constipation.

Adding flaxseed to oatmeal, protein shakes, and smoothies are just a few ways to get more flaxseed into your diet. I love to bake with flaxseed to give my breads and muffins more fiber. Flax is high in both soluble and insoluble fiber, which helps your body with the elimination process. Flax is also low in carbohydrates. According to the Mayo Clinic, most adults should consume between 25-40 grams of fiber every day from foods that are high in fiber. Flax meal is recommended because it's easier to digest than small, hard flaxseed. If you have a coffee grinder, you can use that to grind up flaxseeds. Flaxseeds should be stored in an airtight container in the refrigerator to preserve freshness. Ground flaxseed can be put in yogurt or mixed into sauces like marinara sauce. Be sure to drink a lot of water when adding more fiber to your diet. Fiber helps to keep you feeling full longer, which will help with weight loss or portion control.

Cereals
There are many different choices in the cereal aisle, and many of them are loaded with sugar, artificial colors and flavors, preservatives, and very little nutrition. The best cereal is 100% whole-grain oatmeal that can be prepared in about 10 minutes. It's low in calories, has no sugar, is full of fiber, and helps fight heart disease. Instant oatmeal that is flavored has sugar and artificial ingredients. The original instant oatmeal is a better option, but it lacks the nutrients and fiber of the whole oats.

Boxed breakfast cereals come in all different types and flavors, from Frosted Flakes and Fruit Loops to Raisin Bran. These cereals are full of sugar, artificial color, artificial flavor, and lack fiber and nutrients. These sugary snacks are marketed to children, who love the colors and the catchy jingles in the commercials, but they're not healthy and should be avoided. Some of the healthy brands are Nature's Path, Barbara's, and a few of the store brands that say 100% whole grains and no artificial ingredients, but you need to be careful when choosing from the healthy cereals. Some of the wheat biscuit or oat cereals are unsweetened. Read the label to be sure, and look at the serving size. Remember that a product can say 0 grams of sugar per serving even if it has 0.5 grams of sugar or less per serving. The serving size may be 1/2 cup or 1/4 cup depending on the type of cereal.

The amount of sugar, fat, and number of calories per serving will give you an idea of what's in the cereal. Look at the ingredients to see if there are different types of sugar and if the cereal has granola bits in it. I've noticed some of the flakes of cereal that were low in sugar and 100% whole grains have started putting granola in the cereal, which greatly increases the sugar, fat, and number of calories in each serving. By mixing a healthy cereal with one that has raisins, granola, or other high-calorie fruits and grains in it, the amount of the sugar will be reduced as well as the calories and you still get a little burst of flavor. I like dry cereal that is unsweetened so I can add stevia leaf and unsweetened almond milk, which gives it added flavor.

Any cereal that's low in sugar and high in fiber is good, but few are as good as thick-cut oatmeal that you cook at home. When you eat oatmeal, it helps keep you feeling full because it's high in fiber, and it also lowers blood pressure and helps with the elimination process. Unflavored oatmeal with no sugar added is an effective way to get the fiber the body needs. By adding some fresh berries and stevia leaf, the oatmeal will be naturally sweetened and full of vitamins. This is a smart choice for a quick breakfast in the morning. By making a big pot of oatmeal on Sunday, you can have breakfast already made.

Oatmeal can be stored in the refrigerator for a quick breakfast for up to five days. It only takes one minute in the microwave to heat up a bowl of cooked oatmeal. Adding protein powder gives the oatmeal protein, and slivered almonds or chopped nuts give it healthy fat. This is a nutrient-packed breakfast sure to satisfy everyone, even those craving sweets. Oatmeal is also low in calories, which makes it good for those trying to lose weight and save time in the morning.

Plan your meals and snacks for each day and stick to the healthy eating plan I give you in my book. Eat food in its natural state and eat a lot of organic fruits and vegetables, and especially avoid the "dirty dozen," which are fruits and vegetables most highly sprayed with herbicides, pesticides, and insecticides. Eat 100% whole grains and lean proteins while limiting red meat, pork, and processed meat products like bologna, hot dogs, or salami.

How long does it take to lose weight or get into shape?
People have asked me how many years it takes to get into shape. That depends on the individual and what their goals are. What I can say is that combining healthy eating with exercise is the best way to get in shape, lose weight, increase energy and stamina, and improve health. My book *Healthy Meals in Minutes* goes into detail about what to eat, how to navigate the grocery store to avoid junk foods, and how to lose weight and feel strong. Eating the way I eat, by choosing the healthy meals I recommend, will help to keep your blood sugar from spiking or dropping too low, and help prevent obesity and type 2 diabetes. *Healthy Meals in Minutes* also tells you how to lower cholesterol and high blood pressure. It is important for me to remind you that if you're taking medicine to control your blood sugar, cholesterol, or blood pressure, you need to talk to your doctor. Don't stop taking medication without consulting your physician. Many people who have followed this healthy eating plan have been able to go off medication and maintain a healthy life.

By following a healthy eating plan, your body will get the nutrients it needs and avoid harmful chemicals. Using my healthy eating plan will bring about positive changes in your health. Exercise will create positive changes in your body. The combination of a healthy diet and exercise plan will create positive changes faster. When you do cardiovascular exercise, you burn a lot of calories, increase circulation and blood flow, and condition your heart. Building muscle will help your body burn calories all day long. This is a positive reason for lifting weights. People lose muscle as they age, but this doesn't happen through the seventies, eighties, and beyond when weightlifting and healthy eating are a staple in your life. The loss of muscle slows down the metabolism, which causes weight gain and other health issues. The goal is to stay strong and live a long and healthy life.

The number of calories burned during exercise gives you an idea of how many calories you can eat. Whether you're trying to lose weight, maintain weight, gain muscle, or improve your health, knowing how many calories you need to consume is important. If you eat too many calories, you'll gain weight, and eating too little slows your metabolism down. This doesn't mean you have to count calories. I've made my Healthy Eating Plan so easy that you don't have to count calories. All you do is follow the advice, eat healthy foods, exercise daily, and keep your stress level down. Knowing you're eating foods that are good for you helps reduce stress. Read the nutritional information on packaged foods so you know what you're eating and how many calories, fat, protein, carbohydrates, and sugar are in the product. Reading the label will help you determine whether it's healthy or not.

The body requires calories (food) every day to keep it running and to keep your brain running. The body needs healthy carbohydrates, protein, and healthy fats. If you don't get enough calories, your body will go into starvation mode, which means it will start storing fat and slowing down your metabolism to conserve energy. The minimum number of calories needed for a woman is 1,200, and 1,800 calories per day for a man. Eating less than the minimum number of calories per day will only cause your metabolism to slow down. If you're trying to lose weight, you should eat at least the minimum number of calories per day in the form of lean protein, healthy complex carbohydrates, and healthy fats.

Starting an exercise program will help burn more calories. Gaining more muscle will help burn more calories. It's important to understand that when I say to eat healthy carbohydrates, I'm referring to fruits, vegetables, and 100% whole grains, which are healthy carbohydrates. Many packages of junk and processed foods list carbohydrates on the label. These are not the types of carbohydrates I'm recommending.

Eating a healthy diet with fresh fruits and vegetables will help to add fiber to your diet and help keep the elimination process going smooth while reducing bloating. Lifting weights is another way to reduce unwanted fat. Building muscle, you'll be reducing body fat everywhere in the body. By lifting weights several times a week, your body will start building muscle and losing fat. Combining my healthy eating plan with exercise will prove to be a winning combination in the fight against belly fat.

Exercise is a very important part of my life, and it should be a very important part of your life also. Think of it as your morning cup of coffee or shot of adrenaline. It gets you up and moving, and it gets your blood flowing. Exercise is better than any coffee or pastry in the world. Exercise can be incorporated into any time of your day, but mornings are best. Exercise is a positive way to begin the day, and it sets you up for a happy and healthy day.

Exercising will make you want to eat healthier because it makes you feel so good, and it goes hand in hand with my healthy eating plan. If you put good fuel into your body, you will have more energy and get better results at the gym, running, biking, or whatever type of exercise you decide to do.

A combination of weightlifting and cardiovascular will build lean muscle mass and improve the function of the most important organ, which is your heart. You can lose weight, stop smoking, improve your health, reverse many types of diseases or illnesses, and get off many medications that sedentary people end up on because they don't exercise and eat healthy. Just doing two things can improve your life so much that it could be the difference between life and death. Exercise and healthy eating can literally save your life.

Chapter 6: Where to Begin – Start Now, Exercise

Many people ask me, "When is the best time to start an exercise program?" That's easy. It's right now. Don't wait another day to start an exercise program and eat healthy foods. When people ask me when they should start an exercise program or start eating healthy, I'm always surprised they ask. If your house was on fire, would you ask someone else when you should evacuate? This is something that you need to do now, today and every day from now on. Take care or your body. You only get one body, and it's your responsibility to take care of it. Start right now by making a list of all the healthy foods you need from the store. Buy my book *Healthy Meals in Minutes* and use the list I have in the book. Eliminate all junk foods, fast foods, and processed foods. Eliminate all the unhealthy foods that are in your house. This can be done right now. Don't wait until the perfect time, because it will never come if you keep putting it off. By acting immediately, it empowers you to take the next steps that will lead you to a healthy life and the perfect weight.

Typically, after the holidays, you may be thinking about making a resolution to start your healthy eating plan and start to exercise after the new year. The most common New Year's resolution is to lose weight. Everyone wants to lose the unwanted pounds they gained over the holidays that started October 31 with Halloween candy and kept going straight through the New Year's Eve parties. Now they're at the point where the five pounds they gained turned into 10 pounds and then 20 pounds, and the weight kept piling on year after year.

When people gain weight, many may live in denial. They continue gaining weight and buy stretch pants and bigger sizes and continue to gain weight because they keep doing the things that caused them to gain weight in the first place. Weight gain is a sign that you need to change what you're doing. Getting depressed, upset, and complacent is not the answer. The correct response to gaining weight is to take action to lose the weight you gained. Decide right now that you are going to lose the excess weight and never put it on again. Put on your running shoes and go for a run, jog, or walk, or go to the gym. Any type of workout will make you feel confident and positive. Starting your day with exercise will make you feel good all day long. Congratulate yourself every time you do something that is good for you. Surround yourself with positive people, and keep up with my blogs at tracydwyer.com for healthy and motivational tips.

Starting an exercise program is a matter of planning and execution, which is something that you do every day with your work, family, and chores. Find an hour and a half in your day to exercise and put it on your schedule. You can plan your exercise the same way you prioritize your family events. Take the things that are set, like the time you need to start work or drop the kids off at school, and plan your exercise two hours prior to your first task of the day. If you start the day by watching television, going to get coffee, playing games on the computer, or other nonessential tasks, use that time to do your exercise. This gives you the extra time you need to fit exercise into your busy life.

The best time to exercise is in the morning because if you get up early, there are no distractions. Between the hours of four to seven a.m., there's not much going on, and it's a good time to go to the gym and get a workout in. If your gym doesn't open early in the morning, go for a run or a walk before you go to the gym. Use the gym for weightlifting and muscle-building exercises and the time before the gym opens to do some type of cardiovascular exercise.

What type of person are you?

Have you ever heard of a "weekend warrior?" This is someone who only works out on the weekends. Some weekend warriors do extremely hard workouts on the weekend and nothing else. I'm more interested in striking a balance by integrating exercise into my daily life.

There are many ways to increase your activity level throughout the day. Use the stairs instead of the elevator, and park your car at the end of the parking lot instead of right next to the store. Walk to the park or to school, or ride your bike. I loved living in Campbell, California, because I could ride my bike on the trail that was just a mile from my house. I would take it all the way to Los Gatos Creek Trail, up the face of Lexington Dam. There was a road that went all the way around the dam and through the trees in a loop, and then I would ride back home. It was about a two-and-a-half-hour ride, and it was beautiful. That was something I looked forward to on weekends. Some people work out every day. Any exercise is better than none. If you're not doing any form of exercise, this is a good time to start. What you start with is up to you, but I can tell you that the more days you get an hour of exercise, the better you will feel.

"I've never done any exercise"

If you've never done any exercise, check with your doctor before starting a new exercise program to address any health issues or concerns. It's always best to start slowly and build up instead of jumping into a rigorous workout. Join a gym and consult a professional trainer who can teach you the proper technique for lifting weights. Proper form is very important regardless of the type of exercise you start.

Gyms also have many classes for cardiovascular exercise such as aerobics, cycling, Pilates, yoga, and some have group weightlifting classes. All of these are perfect for beginners, and you can go at your own pace. It's important not to try to keep up with others who have been taking the class for a long time. It will be obvious which people are more experienced, but don't let that bother you. Each person in the gym or in a class has been at the exact place you are now as a beginner. Showing up at the gym is an accomplishment, and everyone there including yourself is there to improve themselves. Some people are more coordinated than others and some are stronger, but everyone is there for the same reason, and that is to get a workout. As you get comfortable with lifting weights or taking classes, you'll get stronger, improve balance, and stamina, and become more coordinated. As a matter of fact, I didn't start going to the gym, lifting weights, or running until I was 35 years old. Before that, it was physical education class for 30 minutes during the school year, and swimming and going to the beach during the summer.

"I don't have time to exercise"

One thing that's equal for everyone is the amount of time we have in a day. There are 24 hours in a day, and it's up to each one of us to use them wisely. Schedule an hour a day for exercise and choose something that is of interest to you or that you can do for an hour.

In the beginning, the duration doesn't have to be a full hour. An hour can be something that you strive and build up to. The hour can be 30 minutes of cardiovascular exercise and 30 minutes of weight training. Any exercise that gets your heart rate up is cardiovascular, such as jumping rope, rowing, elliptical trainer, stair stepper, treadmill, hiking, biking, and aerobics. Dancing is also an effective exercise and is something you can do in a class or at home. Making a conscious decision to exercise is the most important thing you can do along with eating healthy. It doesn't matter how many things you try, as long as you keep exercising. It helps to enjoy what you're doing, but it's not mandatory. There may be an exercise that you don't love but the results are excellent. Exercising may be hard at first, but it will become easier as you build your strength and stamina and a set time to exercise every day.

Finding new ways to fit exercise into your day is something that keeps life interesting. There are many online exercise programs and DVDs that you can use in the comfort of your own home. You must set aside time to exercise every day. Plan at least one hour a day for exercise and stick with your time frame. Making excuses on Monday may keep you from your exercising the next day. Keeping on schedule will help you reach your goal of daily exercise. I commit to daily exercise because it keeps me on track and on schedule. Exercise may vary due to illness, weather, or something else may come up. If this happens, make sure to fit your exercise in later in the day or add some extra exercise the next day, but don't make a habit of missing exercise. When you're feeling tired, push yourself to get out of bed in the morning and get going. Most of the time, when you get to the gym or start whatever exercise you're doing, your energy will pick up and you'll find your rhythm and momentum. When you complete your exercise, you will be happy that you got it done. There's such a feeling of satisfaction when you get through an exercise session. Pat yourself on the back and be happy that you motivated yourself to get your exercise done. The rest of your day will go much better when you start your day with exercise.

"I'm not a morning person"
People who say they aren't morning people may want to sleep in instead of going to the gym. Once you get into a pattern of setting your exercise clothes out in the morning with everything ready to go, it makes it easier for you to get up and exercise. If you can't go in the morning because you have young children at home, create an exercise that you can do at home. Find a place where you can put a spinning bike, weights, and exercise bands. It doesn't take much room to store enough equipment for your daily exercise routine. If you don't have enough room to leave your equipment set up, or if you have little children, store everything in the closet and bring it out when you're ready to use it. Get up an hour or two before the kids and do your exercise. After your exercise, have breakfast and then start your day. This is an effective way to prepare you for the day and get a routine that doesn't get in the way of other activities.

For people who cannot get to the gym or do exercise in the morning I suggest doing it at lunch time or when you are not rushed. Devote your hour and a half to exercise and find something that fits into your schedule. If you need to divide your sessions into two sessions that is fine also as long as you do the second session. If you do not fit the second session in find another way to exercise or another time to fit activity into your day. Many businesses have a gym or a walking trail where you can go on your lunch time or before work. This is a perfect opportunity for you to get your exercise in and to split your workout to a morning walk or run and afternoon lift weights. I love companies that care enough about their employees to put in a gym, par course or walking/running track.

Many companies offer incentives for employees who exercise, which makes perfect sense. They reward people who are working out. Some will even cover part or all of your gym membership. Be sure to ask at your company, and take advantage of this offer. There are many things you can do at the gym to invest in your health. Cardiovascular exercise can be done on the treadmill, where you can walk or run on flat or incline. The elliptical trainer is another piece of equipment that can be used to get your heart rate up, burn a lot of calories, and condition your heart and lungs. There are also stationary bikes and cycling classes. Cycling classes have spinning bikes that can be pedaled while sitting or standing. The instructor plays music and gives you the cues to sit, stand, speed up, and increase the tension on the bike.

Building muscle helps you burn more calories, and what better place to do that other than a gym? There are free weights, weight machines, and weightlifting classes. It is very important to build muscle to support your body and help protect your spine. Muscle helps improve posture and increase your metabolism so you burn more calories all day long. Using exercise bands and stability balls will also increase muscle, strength, and balance.

Adapt your workout

Every location may have something different than what you're used to. I've been to gyms in Europe, Canada, Mexico, and the Caribbean, which were all different. I've learned to be a "traveler" instead of a "tourist." A tourist is one who goes somewhere new and complains about how it isn't like where they're from. A traveler knows not to complain and adapts to wherever they are with a positive attitude. If the cardio room is dark, I bring a little flashlight in my gym bag so I can see. If it's too hot, I bring a personal fan and clip it to the machine I'm working on. I still do my cardio in my jog top without a shirt and put it on when I'm done and ready to start lifting weights. It's important to feel comfortable when working out, wherever you may be. When I was in Montreal, I found a gym and took a Pilates class. When the class started, the instructor was speaking French. I followed along the best I could by watching others. When the instructor realized I didn't understand French, he used English, which was extremely nice, and everyone spoke English and French.

Have confidence

If you go to any gym, track, or running trail, you'll see a variety of body shapes, sizes, ages, and genders. Everyone is there for the same reason, and that is to improve their health, and everyone sweats. When you think about going to the gym or to a track, all you have to worry about is getting there early enough to get a parking spot. Once you're inside, no one is looking at what type of body you have. Sweat is the body's natural cooling system for reducing body temperature, and sweating when you're working out means you're working hard and reaping the benefits of exercise. People also sweat when they're nervous, and for a variety of other reasons. Regardless of the reason, don't be embarrassed about sweating. Remember, you're going to tell yourself that you are amazing, positive, and have a great body. Train your mind to think the best of everyone, especially yourself. Always be good to yourself, especially if you are fortunate and don't have any medical limitations or physical limitations. Put 100% effort into everything you do, and you'll see fast results and instantly feel better just for showing up.

Right clothes, right equipment

Many forms of exercise only require a pair of sports shoes (tennis shoes) for whatever activity you're doing. In places with a mild climate all year long like Southern California, shorts and a tee-shirt are enough. If you live where there are seasons with drastic temperature changes, dress appropriately for the weather outside. The clothes that wick away sweat or that keep you warm in the winter are only needed if you're running, or in temperatures that get very hot, humid, or cold. When you begin working out, especially if you're going to lose weight, wear whatever is comfortable. Don't go out and buy a new wardrobe or expensive workout clothes until you lose the weight. Make the new clothes a reward for losing weight.

Going to a gym isn't mandatory, but it does give you a lot of variety, and the weather won't keep you from working out. If you want to work out at home, there are a few simple things that you can buy. Dumbbells can be used at home and don't take up much room. Buy two of each size, from five to 20 pounds. Men may want to lift heavier weights because they're naturally stronger and have more muscle than women. There are stacks of weights from five to 45 pounds on an A-shaped frame, which doesn't take up much room. A weight bench that can be used flat or on an incline gives you a wide range of exercises. There are also many exercises you can do without a bench. Exercise bands with handles come in a variety of different tensions and can be held in place in the door jamb while you exercise. They're very easy to use and can be stored in a shoe box or the bag they came in. Instructions come with the bands and can also be found online or on a DVD. For more of a challenge, buy a Bosu Ball, which is like a half ball with a flat base to help with stability and balance exercises.

Workout out alone or with others
The best thing about working out alone is you are on your schedule. You don't have to wait for anyone, and you can do whatever you want to do. I looked forward to riding my bike alone on the weekends through the hills of Los Gatos. I used to love to skate alone at the beach when I was in Southern California. There are usually other people out riding their bikes or running on the trails, and there are always people at the gym. Go wherever you want to exercise, and find someone who is working out hard and keep pace with them. Challenge yourself and work hard. You will end up meeting new friends, and if you want a workout partner, they aren't hard to find. Hiring a personal trainer is always an effective way to start by having someone get you through your workout. The fact that you are paying for a session and a trainer is waiting for you will motivate you to stay on schedule. There are like-minded people everywhere who are trying to improve their health by exercising. Introduce yourself, and ask if they'd like to work out with you. People who are working out can be very helpful if you ask them, and they'll be willing to give you some tips.

At the gym, you'll see a variety of people at various fitness levels, and there are many options to choose from when it comes to the type of exercise you can do. Take an aerobics class or a cycling class or use the elliptical trainer or stationary bike. The goal is to get your body moving and your blood flowing.

Classes like cycling or BODYPUMP may look intimidating to someone who has never taken one of these before. Don't let this keep you from attending a class and giving it your all. You're not in competition with anyone but yourself. By this I mean challenge yourself to do a little more or do a little better each time you go to a class or the gym. When you attend a class for the first time, show up 10 minutes early and speak with the instructor to let them know that you're new and may need to be shown some modifications until you can catch up with others in class. Remember that you may not be able to reach the level of some people in the class. There will always be people who have been taking the class for years or are naturally gifted, flexible, or stronger than others. This is something that you know going into the class so you don't overwork, overtrain, or overstretch. A good instructor will walk around or at least look at everyone's form. Keep this in mind with any type of class or group participation activity. Don't miss out on a chance to try something new just because others are more advanced than you are.

Classes at a gym are taught by instructors who teach beginner to advanced classes, which are usually listed for each class. I attended a yoga class at a new gym and talked to the instructor before the class to let her know I might need modifications. The class wasn't listed as advanced, but it was. The instructor didn't give any modifications, so I had to do some stretching and yoga poses I already knew. Pushing yourself or overstretching can cause serious injuries, and that was the last thing I needed. She didn't like me doing different poses, but I didn't want to hurt myself or waste my time by leaving her class. Even in cycling classes, the instructor gives cues to people who can't keep up or need a slower, easier pace. Be sure to speak up if this happens to you. For the most part, instructors are very nice and willing to help newcomers. Most of them will ask at the beginning of the class if there are any people new to whatever they're teaching. This will make your class more enjoyable for you and the instructor.

When you're around people who are working out and eating healthy, it makes you want to follow their example. It's infectious. You see people biking, running, and lifting weights at the gym, and it motivates you to do the same. Find the people who are working out hard and look like they're enjoying their exercises, and imitate them. This is especially important for people who have never worked out before or who are having trouble getting started. If you watch other people working out, enjoying themselves, and showing results, you'll want to do the same.

Be inspired by others, and be an inspiration to others. Everyone has to start somewhere. No one wakes up looking trim and strong; they must work at it. A friend from my gym started dating a man who didn't work out. He wanted her to stay home with him instead of going to the gym in the morning. Her response was, "Do you think I just wake up looking like this?" When she told me, I laughed hard and encouraged her to get him to work out with her. Once he started going to the gym with her, they were both happy and healthy. It's helpful to work out with your significant other or a friend, but if you don't have anyone, go to the gym and be around people with the same goals as you. Even if you don't know anyone, it'll feel like you're among friends. If you go at the same time every day, you'll see the same people every day and make some friends. Even if they're only gym friends, they're still there with you every morning working out, and that is a powerful motivation.

There are a variety of classes like Zumba, BODYPUMP, cycling, Pilates, and yoga. Cycling classes are challenging and good for burning calories while having fun. The tension can be turned up to make it harder to pedal, just like riding a bike up a hill, and you can stand and pedal. The instructor will play music and give you the cues for the cadence and tell you when the hills are coming up, which means turn up the tension. When I lived in California, I took many classes, and they were all fun.

When we moved to Fort Hood, Texas, they didn't have cycling classes at the local gym. I couldn't run every day as I had in California because of the weather, so I bought a spinning bike for my house. I now have two spinning bikes—one for me, and one for my husband. We use them on the weekends and then go to the gym. During the week, we use the elliptical trainer for cardiovascular exercise and then lift weights. It's wonderful to have someone to work out with. No matter where we are, we find a gym and work out.

It's important to lift weights to keep your muscles strong to support your body. More muscle means more calories are being burned. The more muscle you have, the easier it is to lose weight. When you gain muscle, you will look and feel better. Your weight may go up on the scale, but if you're gaining muscle and not gaining fat, it's fine. Your clothes will fit better when you lose the fat because the muscle takes up less room. You will also be able to eat more food without getting fat if you eat right and do cardiovascular exercise and weight training. Doing one or the other will reduce weight, but the combination will give you faster results.

The freedom you feel from being physically fit is like no other. The best days of my life were when I went running in the hills at Rancho San Antonio in Los Altos. This beautiful wildlife preserve was my favorite place to run because of the dirt trails with hills and the wildlife all around. There is nothing like a morning run before work. Running is a fabulous form of exercise, and it will get you in shape fast. Different ways of approaching exercise and finding what you love are important to keep you on a daily exercise routine. You can take one day off a week if you're training hard and eating right. If you do moderate exercise and have no injuries, it's okay to work out every day.

It's important to warm up and stretch before and after exercise. This can be done by learning how to stretch the muscles you're going to use. One effective way to stretch and improve flexibility is yoga. Yoga helps with flexibility, strength, and stability, and it calms the mind. It also teaches you to breathe. Breathing is important for your body. Yoga connects mind, body, and soul. It gets you in touch with your body and your breathing and helps you to relax into the poses.

Rest and recovery play a big part in your overall health and are very important aspects of your daily life. When you don't get enough rest, problems will start creeping up and may become serious issues. No matter what you're doing, your body is constantly working, moving, and burning calories.

Chapter 7: Exercise is a Gift

Every part of the body is made to move, become strong, and meet whatever challenge there is. A baby will learn to move, roll, pullup, crawl, climb, and walk within 10-18 months. A baby starts exercising at birth when they cry and move their bodies. The momentum continues as they grow and learn to run, play games, ride a bike, roller skate and play sports.

When children run and play, they don't realize they're exercising while having fun. Exercise is fun! Whether you're young or old, everyone needs to exercise. Exercise is not something you do occasionally; it's something you need to do every day. Exercise keeps you feeling healthy, young, and fit. It's not just about how you look. It's also about how you feel. Exercise brings joy to your life because it increases blood flow throughout the body. Cardiovascular exercise will keep your heart strong and burn a lot of calories. Lifting weights will build muscles, which will help you burn calories throughout the day.

Doing a combination of cardiovascular exercise and weight training is a winning combination. This doesn't mean you have to go to the gym every day, but think of the advantages of daily exercise. It keeps you feeling and looking young, and at the same time, you'll be able to do more of the things in life that healthy people do, like run in a race, play with your children and grandchildren, and have fun.

Getting up early in the morning and going to the gym or going on a run, a bike ride, or a brisk walk is the best way to start the day. Make it a point to do some form of exercise every day. There are so many types of exercise that it will be easy to find a program you can stick to. Exercise is not a chore; it is a GIFT. Good health is a gift you can give yourself and your family. Exercise is something you can teach your children do. Take a fun family hike or a family bike ride. Go for a walk and enjoy nature. Most people can walk or use the stairs instead of taking the elevator. Fit exercise in whenever possible. Many people use fitbits or some type of step counter to motivate them to move their bodies. Knowing you are improving your health should be a powerful motivator.

Walking programs
Starting a walking program is very simple way to work into an exercise program. Walking can be done from your home, at a track, or on a treadmill at the gym. A brisk walk can get you blood circulating and may be the perfect place to start if you haven't done any type of exercise. There is usually a smooth transition from a brisk walk to a walk-run. This is just what it sounds like. Walk for a few minutes and then run for however long you can. It doesn't have to be a fast run. It can be a little jog. This is a way of conditioning the body for more vigorous exercise.

I've known many people who have dropped a lot of pounds just by walking. My neighbor in Texas was scheduled for knee surgery. The fear of surgery motivated her to start walking every morning. She walked a little farther and a little faster each time and lost over 100 pounds. Her knee stopped hurting, and she no longer needed the surgery. The extra weight she was carrying was putting stress on her knee. By losing weight and getting stronger, she was able to avoid surgery.

Cardiovascular exercise

There is one muscle that you need to keep running strong, and that is your heart. Cardiovascular exercise keeps your heart and lungs in shape. Cardiovascular exercise is any exercise that gets you into your heart rate training zone. Unlike weightlifting, cardio gets your heart rate elevated for a duration of time. There are many ways to get your heart rate up to condition your heart and lungs. Cardio machines at the gym usually have a built-in monitor, which is not as accurate as wearing your own, but it gives you an idea of the number of calories you burn during your exercise. Try for an hour of cardiovascular exercise a day and see how far you can get. In the beginning, the session may only be 20 minutes, and then each session adds five or 10 minutes until you get up to an hour. If you're doing cardio and weights in the same session, you may have an hour and a half to work out, so divide your time into 50 minutes of cardio and 40 minutes of weights, or one hour of cardio and 30 minutes of weights.

Cardiovascular exercise burns more calories per hour than weightlifting and is an effective way to burn calories and stored fat. By keeping the heart rate elevated for a sustained amount of time, the heart is being conditioned along with the lungs to work more efficiently. This improves stamina, energy, circulation, and helps prevents obesity, high cholesterol, high blood pressure, heart disease, diabetes, and cancer. Effective forms of cardio exercise are running, biking, skating, swimming, elliptical trainer, spin bike, and treadmill with elevation. Anything that keeps your heart rate up for a sustained time is ideal. This is the most important muscle in the body, so take care of it by doing cardiovascular exercise.

Spinning bikes are used for cardiovascular exercise because they get your heart rate up quickly and in a fun way. Taking spinning or cycling classes at the gym is always fun and challenging. Buy a spinning bike for your home and ride it while you watch a concert or movie on your TV. Listen to fast-paced music and challenge yourself by doing fast intervals followed by slow intervals with more resistance. These bikes allow you to sit or stand while pedaling. They also have a tension knob to increase or decrease the tension, making it harder or easier to pedal. This is a wonderful way to get a combination of cardiovascular exercise for your heart and build strength in your legs at the same time. The primary muscles used when spinning are the quadriceps muscles, which are located at the front top part of your leg, and the gluteus muscle, or your rear end. Indoor cycling burns calories at a high rate and will burn excess fat. Your legs and gluteus will become toned and lean, and you will release those feel-good hormones called endorphins, which come from getting a good workout. These bikes are convenient for working out at home whenever you want. They don't take up much room and have wheels on the front so they can be placed anywhere with ease. I love having my spinning bike for times when I can't make it to the gym because I have an early meeting or simply to change up my workout.

Most spinning bikes come with an instructional DVD, or you can buy them, stream, or go to YouTube and find a spinning class. If you've ever been to a spinning class at a gym and already know how to use your spinning bike, all you need is some music, and away you go. When I ride my spinning bike at home, I love to find a great band playing in concert. Use your DVR to record a concert, dance show, or anything that plays music with a good fast-paced beat. When the music is slower, you can turn up the tension and pedal at a slower, harder pace. When the music is fast, turn down the tension and pedal faster, or switch to medium tension and pedal standing up. Any combination of speed, tension, standing, and sitting can be used. You are in control of your very own spinning class. It's fun to challenge yourself and hear some good music at the same time.

I don't endorse any websites or spinning coaches or instructors. Finding a qualified instructor online is an option you can explore on your own, but I recommend you do it ahead of time so that when it's time to do your workout, everything will be ready to go. These endurance coaching sessions can give you the motivation and instruction if you want to have a coach training you in your own home. These can be found on-demand, streaming, or on YouTube. If you've never taken a spinning class and need help, I recommend going to a spinning class in person and taking a few classes. Let the instructor know you're new so they can help you adjust the bike and make suggestions.

Spinning bikes offer a low-impact workout with high intensity while you burn fat and calories. Finding a spinning bike is easy if you go to a gym or a store that sells spinning bikes and test one out. The most expensive bike is not always the best bike. The cheap bikes will be a waste of money because they may be wobbly and not run smoothly. Both of my bikes are Star Trac; one is a home bike and the other is a bike used by gyms. Both bikes work well, and my husband and I use them all the time. This is a bike that doesn't have any electronics or screens. It's a pure spinning bike, and we usually find a fast-paced concert or something with music that keeps us motivated for an hour. I don't like to watch TV shows or movies when working out because I want to concentrate on my workout. Building strength and endurance is always my goal when working out.

Spinning bikes have wheels on the front so they can be placed wherever you want to use them. I store mine in my sunroom and move them to the living room when I work out so I can listen to my music show. Then we roll them back to the sunroom where they fit nicely in the corner. This is one of the best pieces of equipment I have ever purchased for my home. When I can't get to the gym or it's closed, I can still get a workout at home.

Equipment

Home gyms come in handy when you're pressed for time or if you have kids at home. Bands with handles come in a variety of weights, resistance, and they come with a strap that goes under the door to hold them in place. The handles will both be on your side of the door, and there are many exercises you can do with resistance bands for your legs, upper body, arms, and core. They usually come with instructions, or you can look online for information and exercises. One important thing to remember when using resistance bands is to make sure the door opens away from you, which will keep you from getting hit if it opens.

Dumbbells are a good inclusion to your home gym, and a bench or an exercise step will give you a wide variety of exercises to do, either standing or on the bench. Depending on your ability, you can buy different weights. There are charts you can buy with diagrams of exercises for each body part on them, and there are workout DVDs, online information, and classes. You can also hire a trainer or sign up at a gym to work out with a trainer who can teach you proper techniques to strengthen various muscle groups and avoid injury. After learning the proper techniques, you will be able to work out on your own, at the gym or at home.

I have sets of eight, 10, 12, and 20-pound dumbbells at my house, and I have a step that I use as a bench. This step and the weights can be put in a closet when I'm not using them, or when kids come to my house. If you drop any size wight on a toe or foot, it will hurt, especially a child.

Having exercise equipment at home makes it easy to get a full workout any time of the day. This makes it easy to get a workout in before the children wake up, and then you're ready for them when they get up. Schedule a 60 or a 90-minute workout if you're doing weights and cardiovascular exercise at the same time. If you're unable to get it all done at one time, work out two times a day. Divide your workout into cardiovascular exercise in the morning and weights in the afternoon, or vice versa. Run, walk, or spin in the morning, and lift weights in the afternoon at home or at the gym. When you have equipment at your house, it's easy to get your workout in every day.

Music

One of the best ways to transport yourself to another place is by listening to music. A large variety of music can be accessed on your computer, mobile device, cell phone, and car radio. Music can put you in a good mood, make you feel relaxed, or give you the energy to get through your workout. Different types of music can be used for evoking different emotions, which makes music a perfect choice for many situations.

There are many different genres of music and many reasons for choosing certain music. The choices of music you listen to may be made because you like the genre of music, the beat of the music, or the group or person creating the music. Many times, you listen to music playing in the background of a movie. During a massage, soothing music will be played to help you relax and release tension in your body.

The fact is, music is a big part of life, and it makes sense when you realize how much it works to create a certain feeling or mood.

Create a playlist of music from a variety of genres and have it available so you can listen to whatever music complements what you're doing. Music that's fast-paced with a catchy beat works well for cardiovascular exercise at the gym but can also be motivating when you're at home doing housework. When it's time to wrap up your day or cook dinner, find music that's slow with a softer beat that helps you unwind. When it's time to get ready for bed, listen to relaxing music that calms the mind. There is music specifically created to help you relax and go to sleep, which is very beneficial if you have trouble turning off your mind. Music is a tool to use any time you want to change your mood or motivate yourself. Have fun creating a variety of music to listen to as you go through your day.

Exercise journal and monitor
One way to track your exercise progress is by writing it down in an exercise journal and wearing a heart rate monitor during exercise. By writing down your daily exercise and what you eat, it's easy to track the progress you make each day and where you may need to make changes. For years, I've been using my exercise journal, which I detail in my book *Healthy Meals in Minutes*. The body burns a greater amount of fat during lower-intensity cardiovascular exercise over a longer duration than it does during higher intensity. My monitor tracks cardiovascular exercise, such as using the elliptical trainer or treadmill, and tells me the duration, average heart rate, time in my fat-burning zone, time above the zone, time below the zone, the number of calories I burn, and the percentage of fat calories I burn during my cardiovascular exercise.

When I lift weights, I use my monitor to tell me the same information, so I know the total calories burned during my workouts. Most days, I do cardiovascular exercise before lifting weights. If you're exercising, it's good to warm up before you begin lifting weights. Some people like to lift weights one day and do cardiovascular exercise the next. Sometimes, I lift weights first and then do cardiovascular exercise. The goal is to do both types of exercise to improve your overall health. Cardiovascular exercise will increase blood circulation throughout the body, and it will burn more calories during exercise. Building muscle helps your body burn more calories all day long. Both will greatly benefit your body. High-intensity exercise releases endorphins, the feel-good hormones, and it fights stress hormones such as adrenaline and cortisol. Endorphins are the body's natural mood elevator and pain reliever.

I like to use a heart rate monitor when I'm walking to keep track of my calories burned and my heart rate. It's fun to see the difference between the number of calories burned on the elliptical trainer and walking. When I had surgery, I used walking as my exercise during recovery. Normally, I burn between 450 and 525 calories during an hour of cardiovascular exercise. Walking, I would maybe burn 150-200 calories in an hour. It was important for me to stick to my healthy eating plan and to walk three times a day. In the beginning, I could only walk about 20 minutes at a time. As I was feeling better, I increased the duration. If I started feeling any pain, I would rest and then go back to walking later or the next day.

Hiking
You can get outside and enjoy nature by hiking on trails in parks or in the mountains. Hiking has various levels, from easy to advanced, with hills and flats that'll get your heart rate up and burn calories while you enjoy nature. There are different hiking trails for

those of different abilities, making it easy for everyone to enjoy. Jerry and I hiked the Grand Canyon when we were in Arizona, which I highly recommend. It's breathtakingly beautiful. There are many trails to hike, and people can take the trail that meets their abilities. We also hiked to the top of Mount Tallac in Lake Tahoe, which is 9,738 feet above sea level. It was my first time hiking a mountain, and I was a bit nervous even though Jerry had climbed many mountains with groups of people using ropes, crampons, picks, and other climbing tools. They also slept overnight on the way up the mountain. The thought of sleeping in the cold on the side of a mountain was a bit scary. Luckily, we were going to be walking on a trail that winds around the mountain on an incline, which makes it easier than climbing up the side of a mountain. When we reached the top, we looked over Lake Tahoe, and the view was beautiful. We brought lunch and ate at the peak of the mountain. I always loved running, but hiking is a very different experience, and looking down to the bottom of the mountain where we started gave me an amazing sense of accomplishment. There are websites that tell you where the trails are in your local area. I recommend taking a lunch and exploring a new place everywhere you go.

Running outside

Running outside is another effective way to get exercise and enjoy nature. Even if you're in the city, there's always something to enjoy while running. Make sure to run facing traffic, and be on the sidewalk or someplace safe from cars. Running on a track is a safe place to run, especially if you're just starting to run for the first time. Many tracks have a rubbery surface that's easier on the body than cement. If you have a paved trail where you can run without worrying about cars, all the better. I used to love running at Rancho

San Antonio in Los Altos. It's a beautiful wildlife preserve that's all dirt and has many trails to run on. There are rocks, tree roots, and wild animals, which are all part of the experience and really brings nature into your run. Many wildlife preserves don't have any lights, so going before sunup means you'll need a flashlight to be able to see the trails. Many nature trails close at dusk for safety reasons.

I always loved going for a run when the sun was coming up. Some of the best and most spiritual times of my life were spent running at Rancho San Antonio. There are many trails that go up to the top of the hills and some that go down into the valleys. One of the trails is a very long, steep run that leads to the top, where you can see the entire city from San Jose to Milpitas, including Moffett Field, which was an army base in Mountain View. I could even see the bridges in San Francisco. It's a wonderful place to run, hike, or just walk. I ran all the different trails and gave them my own names. One of my runs was eight miles up the hill to a flat patch of trail and then into a meadow. I called this the eight-mile tree run. It took a little over an hour to do the loop. All the runs started at the main parking lot and past some small bushes and a field. Many times, we would see wild turkey, deer, and even bobcats. The bobcats we saw were very young, so they weren't too scary.

One morning, I was running alone and was high on the trail, and I could see a cat in the distance. I was far from it, but as I got closer, I could tell it was a mountain lion, and he was not afraid of me. I walked slowly backwards and held my shirt up in the air— the thing to do when you see a mountain lion is to make yourself look big. When I got a safe distance from him and he wasn't following me, I ran as fast as I could down the hill and didn't stop until I was in the parking lot. This happened one time in all the years I ran there. I went running there on the weekends and a day or two during the week if I had time before work. It was a very inspiring time for me. I had a lot to be thankful for. I survived colon cancer in 1994, and that was when I started running. I loved running in the hills so much that I continued running at Rancho San Antonio for nine years.

Weightlifting

Many people associate muscle mass with bodybuilding, and big bulging muscles that only bodybuilders possess. This could not be further from the truth when it comes to health, preventing injuries, and losing weight. The more muscle mass you have, the more calories you burn all day long, even when not working out. Think about what your body does without you telling it to do. The heart is pumping blood, the kidneys and liver are filtering, the stomach is digesting the food you eat, and the bowels are working to eliminate the food not used by the body. The calories you eat that aren't used up are stored as fat to be used later.

The more muscle you have, the more calories you'll burn, and the more calories you can consume without gaining weight or unwanted body fat. Lean muscle mass is more compact than fat, so your body will be tighter and leaner when you develop more muscle. Cardiovascular exercise burns a lot of calories, but muscle continues to burn calories all day long. To build and maintain muscle mass, you'll need to eat enough calories. Imagine being able to eat more and not worry about gaining weight, which is what muscle mass will do for you.

One of the best reasons to do exercise that builds muscle, such as lifting weights, is the muscles around your skeleton are holding you up, carrying your body around, getting you up and down the stairs, and taking excess pressure off your back, knees, and joints.

Muscle is needed to prevent injury to the body. Muscle can prevent serious injury when you fall or get into an accident. Muscle gives you a protective layer that's harder to penetrate. Think of muscle as an insurance policy that protects your body. The stronger you are, the easier it is to recover from injury. Health and fitness go hand in hand, and taking care of your body by eating healthy foods and exercising daily is the best way to prevent illness.

Men lift weights to build lean muscle mass and to look good, feel strong, and challenge themselves. It's not hard to get a man to lift weights, especially if he's seen the physique that can be achieved.

For women, lifting weights comes with a preconceived notion that they'll get big muscles like a man, and they don't want to be that muscular. Rest assured, you will not develop large muscles. Women don't have the genetic makeup to build large muscles unless they work hard at it, like female bodybuilders, or unless they use enhancement drugs like steroids. Growth hormone and testosterone also help build more muscle, but women don't have as much muscle as men or have the amount of testosterone men possess. Having more muscle and male hormones makes it easier to build muscle and is also why men can lose weight easier and faster than women.

As we age, our bodies begin to put on more fat, lose muscle, and hormones begin to decline. The metabolism begins to slow down, and it gets harder to lose or maintain a healthy weight. But no matter what age you are, you can always build muscle and increase stamina by working out.

Throughout life, exercise can help you maintain muscle, strength, and improve your health. There is never a time when you need to stop exercise due to age. Those who exercise throughout their lives live longer and are happier. As many people will tell you, they don't want to slow down—they want to stay active because it makes them feel and look younger.

For those who have never lifted weights, start with light weights and increase the weight as you get comfortable with the movements. Use a professional trainer or someone who is experienced at lifting weights. By going to a gym and asking for help, you can learn which machines to use and what exercises to do.

Dividing your workout into upper body one day and lower body the next day, and alternating through the week, is a good way to get started. This keeps you from overusing your muscles when you begin to work out. There are many ways to structure daily workouts depending on what you're trying to achieve. Working two muscle groups each day keeps you from overworking any one group of muscles.

Begin with weights that are easy enough to lift with resistance, but not so heavy that they're too hard to do three sets of each exercise with 12 repetitions. Choose three different exercises for each muscle group. You can alternate muscle groups back and forth through the three sets of 12, then move on to the next two exercises and do the same. Be sure to breathe in and out during your sets, and don't hold your breath. If the weights are so heavy that you can't breathe, you should go to lighter weights. Remember, you don't want to be so sore that you have to take the next day off. The goal is to work out every day by doing just enough to feel the burn without overworking the muscles. Never work to the point of pain. This will risk injury, and that's not what should happen when you're beginning to work out. Being a bit sore the next day is normal, but feeling pain at the time of the exercise means you need lighter weight or to do a different exercise.

Weightlifting at any age

Weightlifting and weight-bearing exercises will increase your muscle mass, which helps you burn fat even while at rest. The more muscle mass you have, the more calories you will burn. If you've never lifted weights before, ask a trainer at the gym to help you design a routine. When you join a gym, a trainer will usually show you around the gym and will help you create a routine to strengthen different muscle groups. During the aging process, muscle will be lost, so you must stay active and lift weights. This will greatly reduce the loss of muscle due to aging.

Researchers found that people in their eighties who started a weightlifting routine for the first time were able to gain muscle mass and improve their overall health. Around puberty, kids can start lifting weights. Make sure they're taught proper form from a professional trainer to prevent them from using the wrong technique. This also enables them to understand what muscles they are using to do the exercise. It's important to have good technique to avoid injury. Kids from nine to 12 can be taught to use resistance bands. This should also be something that an experienced person teaches them. There is no age limit on exercise or lifting weights unless your physician tells you to stop due to injury or medical condition. Be sure to consult your physician if you have questions or before starting an exercise program, especially if you have a chronic medical condition.

Muscle fatigue

When muscles fatigue and you feel like you can't do another rep, it's important to recognize the difference between fatigue and strain. Fatigue can be worked through, or you can simply move to a different exercise. Stop and stretch the muscle and move to the next exercise or rest for a few minutes. Strain is something that should be avoided, especially if there is also associated pain. This is a time when you should stop using that muscle to avoid injury. Only you know when you've done enough. Don't let someone tell you to push through the pain. That leads to possible injury and a lengthy period of recovery, which is not the goal. Daily exercise and a lifetime of fitness is the goal.

Sore muscles
Delayed Onset Soreness, or DONS, happens when you push yourself too hard. You may feel good during the workout but later feel very sore, maybe even to the point of pain. This is a good time to take care of yourself and learn to check in with your body. Try stretching, Epsom salt baths, or massage to see if this makes you feel better. When the soreness doesn't subside with any type of therapy or self-care, take the day off and apply the RICE method: Rest, Ice, Compression, and Elevate. This will evaluate the soreness to determine if it's just sore muscles or an injury. For pain in the leg, knee, or shoulder, elevate higher than your heart by lying down and using a pillow to prop up the leg. For upper-body pain, elevate the upper body and use ice. For injury, the best thing to use is ice. After a day or two, you can use heat. Ice relieves swelling and inflammation, and heat relaxes the muscles. Many people would rather use heat, but at the onset of an injury, ice is best. For pain and swelling that doesn't resolve with RICE, see a medical doctor. Sore muscles will feel better after doing the above and taking a day or two off working out.

Creative counting is something I use to keep pushing through my exercise when it's tough, or to make it seem like I have less to do. Instead of counting from one to 12, I count three reps of four, two reps of six, four reps of three, and so on. Break it down however you want to get through your routine. If you're working with time or cardio, divide one hour into 15 minutes, 20 minutes, or 30 minutes until you get to the hour. This helps you achieve mini-goals that you can congratulate yourself for keeping you motivated and making the session go by faster.

Summary

Try different types of exercise that make you feel like a kid again. Have fun, and don't look at exercise like it's some difficult chore. Based on my lifetime of experience, exercise is not a chore, it's a gift, and it's fun!

Chapter 8: My Experience with Exercise

I was born and raised in Southern California, and I loved Hermosa Beach from the time I was a baby. I remember walking across the hot sand and thinking the water was so far away. Now when I go there, it seems so much closer. The beach will always be my favorite place to be. Bodysurfing, surfing, roller skating or rollerblading, bike riding, skateboarding, running, walking, and hiking are all activities that can be done at the beach. It doesn't matter where I travel; I always find a place to exercise. I find walking trails or hiking trails, a gym, or I work out in my room with exercise bands. I love to get up in the morning before the sun comes up and get my exercise in for the day. After exercising, the rest of the day is brighter and I feel happier. When I don't exercise, I feel cranky and sluggish. It's always best to start the day with exercise.

Exercise for me was mostly during the summer because I had school, homework, babysitting my brothers, and doing housework for my mom. There were no organized sports like they have now for girls when I was in grade school. In the summer, there was a girls' softball team in junior high, and I started playing in seventh grade. I remember a day in my sophomore year when I was wearing an outfit from the year before, and the shorts were tight on me. One of the boys in my class said, "You really filled out over the summer." I was so embarrassed and became self-conscious about my weight. Puberty brings changes in the body, which can make one wonder how to stop it. This was a perfect time to learn about food and exercise.

When I was a junior in high school, I went to the beach in the summer and rode my bike to the beach to bodysurf . During the winter months, I ice skated on the weekends or went bowling. Formal team sports started in high school with the Girls' Athletic Association (GAA), and I made the junior-senior team when I was a freshman. We played basketball, flag football, softball, and volleyball. The YMCA had a gymnastics class that I joined in my junior year, and I started gymnastics at my new high school and made the gymnastics team. All the other girls had been taking gymnastics since they were little. I competed in floor exercise, vaulting, and balance beam. I was very flexible and strong, but not at the level of the other girls who had been taking gymnastics since they were small. This would probably be my only year of gymnastics, so I did my best and even won competitions on the balance beam. I used my balance and flexibility to my advantage. Luckily, gymnastics was not as difficult as it is now, or I probably wouldn't have made the team. What is being done on the balance beam now is extraordinary and very difficult. Using the skills I developed proved I could succeed, and that was the important part.

My senior year was filled with difficult chemistry and biology classes so I could get a scholarship to Pepperdine University in Malibu as a premed student so I could reach my dream of becoming a doctor. For that scholarship, I had to get straight A's and change schools in my senior year so I could take the classes I needed. The letter of acceptance came along with my full scholarship. This story will continue in my next book about the business I started in Los Angeles after I graduated.

In 1991, I moved to San Jose in Northern California, which was a big culture and weather shock. The beaches of Southern California had always been a place of joy for me. The beach cured everything from acne to a broken heart. This was also the best place to exercise. Everything from swimming, bodysurfing, surfing, roller skating, bike riding, and walking on the strand was fun in the sun. The big change to riding a bike on the trail in San Jose and Los Gatos was hard for me.

The first thing I learned when I went out on the trail in my bikini to roller skate was that people in San Jose don't skate in bathing suits like they do at the beach in Southern California. People were looking, wondering why I was wearing a bathing suit. It took a little time for me to figure out how I could still exercise outside. Wearing the right clothes for the weather was the key. I am a Southern California native who loves good weather, and it was hard to get used to the colder winters and rain in San Jose. The ocean was an hour's drive, and the water was cold. Riding a bike outside was hard in the winter because it was too cold for my hands and fingers. Gloves, warm pants, and long sleeves helped me get outside in the colder weather.

The grocery store had some cards for a 30-day free gym membership, and I decided to give the gym a try for the first time in my life. When I was at the gym, the weather didn't matter. At 35, I started going to the gym to take aerobic classes and lift weights. Before that time, I never dreamed of lifting weights. The trainer at the gym showed me how to lift weights and gave me an easy routine. Everything else I learned about weightlifting I learned from watching people and taking classes at the gym. The results I got made me stronger, leaner, and gave me more stamina.

Life has its twists and turns, and sometimes it throws you a major curveball. In 1994, I was diagnosed with colon cancer, and I was unsure what would happen. I had already started eating a healthy diet and was exercising daily, but this diagnosis led to me cutting out everything that had any artificial ingredients, sweeteners, preservatives, pesticides, or herbicides. I already had an exercise program, but I kicked it into high gear so I would be strong before surgery, which would be in one month.

Exercise also greatly reduced the stress, along with eating healthy, praying, and going to church. I asked everyone I knew to pray for me and to put me on their prayer list at their church. I read books by all the greatest motivational speakers and read the Bible every day, and spending time with my son was very important. I made sure he knew I was going to be fine. A month after the diagnosis, I had major surgery to remove 10 inches of my colon to make sure it had not spread to any vital organs. The surgery involved an incision from navel to pubic bone. I didn't want my abdominal muscle to be cut open, but the doctor told me that was the only way to make sure the cancer didn't spread.

When I started to wake up after surgery, I thought I was dreaming that people were bringing in beautiful flowers. I was squeezing my mom's hand when I woke up, and I told her about my dream, and she pointed to the room and said, "That was not a dream. Look at all the flowers and cards."

I knew that my biopsy was going to come back negative because that was all I focused on from the time of my diagnosis. My doctor came in and told me the more I got up and walked, the faster I would heal. When the nurses came in to get me up, I stood and got

dizzy, and they said that was enough for the day. My goal was to walk further every day until I made it over to the other side of the hospital where the newborn babies were. Every morning, my mom and dad would come to the hospital and hold my arms while we walked down the hallway. By the end of the week, I made it to see the newborn babies.

From the time I got home, I was determined to walk three times a day and walk a little further every day. My mom stayed an extra week to help me and take care of my son because I couldn't lift, bend, stoop, or open anything. With the incisions down my entire abdomen and inside where they reattached my colon, I couldn't take a chance of anything coming apart. After dropping my son off at school, we would start our walks. Three short walks each day, going a little farther every time. My goal was to make it five blocks to Baskin-Robbins to get a frozen yogurt. By midweek, we walked the distance to the yogurt shop and sat down to eat. Every little move gave me severe pain, but I was determined to keep walking and not take any pain medication. The pain was so severe that it hurt to roll over in bed, stand up, sit down, cough, sneeze, or laugh. Medication would delay healing and make it harder for my bowels to start working again.

I had been through many bad things in my short 36 years, but being told I had cancer was the worst. I would do everything I could to make sure I stayed healthy. My determination, positive thinking, and focus on staying healthy helped me beat cancer. The question I had was how did I get colon cancer? Was it from artificial sweeteners? Was it from stress?

I had a great deal of stress my entire life. What I figured out was that taking the best care of my body from this point on would keep me from ever getting cancer or any other type of disease. I swore I would never have any surgery again. After eight weeks of walking every day and eating healthy, I was released to go back to teaching physical education, and I started my traveling notary public service where I was doing the closing paperwork for refinancing agreements.

There's nothing to stop anyone from achieving what they want in life. Ask yourself, if you could do anything in life without failing, what would it be? Picture yourself doing it, and focus on your success and how it makes you feel. Then live each day with that feeling, and go out and achieve it all. Nothing is holding you back but the excuses you give yourself. Worrying or overthinking is a waste of time. Just get out and do it, and then do the next thing and never give up a chance to try something new.

Not knowing what to do or where to start can keep you in limbo. Just go out and do something. Know that you cannot fail. Put 100% effort into everything you do, and you will never be a failure. Do you know Thomas Edison failed over a thousand times to make a light bulb? On the next try, it worked. If he gave up on the first try, he would have failed. All those failures taught him what he needed to do next. It doesn't matter what you're doing, so long as you're moving forward.

Two months after recovering from having colon cancer and a colon resection, I met a woman at a park in Los Gatos who told me about a race called The Dammit Run. It was a very popular race that was coming up in four weeks, and she suggested I run in it. I told her I was not a runner. She said, "Well, you have a month to train." I had been doing aerobics, step aerobics, and lifting light weights at the gym, but this was a race running through the hills of Los Gatos. I thought that since I had just beat cancer, which most people die from, this would be a great way to prove to myself that I was back and unstoppable. The Dammit Run starts at the high school with one lap around the track, onto the dirt trail up a steep hill, then flat until the hill going up the face of Lexington Dam, then a steep hill and down the other side, and finally back to the school with one more lap around the track.

The next day, I went to the gym and did my normal recovery workout. At lunch, I went to the hills of Los Gatos to take my first run. It was more of a walk with a lot of short runs. This was obviously harder than step aerobics. I was able to run up the first hill at a very slow pace. I did a slow run on the flat part. When I got to the big hill, it was so steep that I had to walk up the whole way. Running down the hill was steep and there were a lot of rocks, but I made it to the bottom and walked the rest of the way to my car. Even though I didn't run the entire way, I loved the feeling of freedom and the satisfaction of making it around the loop through the hills. Since I had beat the colon cancer, the number-two cancer killer of both men and women, I was determined to accomplish the run.

Every other day at lunch, I headed for the hills to do my run with walk breaks. My goal was to do a little more running each time until I got to the point where I could run the flats and walk all the hills. It took me a few weeks to make it all the way around without stopping. Being outside and enjoying the fresh air made it a wonderful experience. Every time I got to the end of the trail, I felt fabulous. The mantras, positive thinking, and visualization helped me achieve my goal of running the entire loop. I never ran the entire distance before the race because the track was unavailable while the school was in session the week of the race. My goal was to run the entire distance and not worry about how long it took me to finish.

On the day of the race, I remember my heart racing with excitement. I had never run in a race in my whole life and now, at 36 years old, I was running in not just any race but a race with three hills and a bunch of very young, fit people. I didn't know the rules of running in a race. I got in the front line with the runners so I could get the full experience of starting on the starting line. When the starter's pistol went off, I started running. Tears welled up in my eyes, but I had to fight the urge to cry. I wiped my eyes and ran my loop around the school, and then we started up to the dirt trail. People were passing me on the left and the right, but that didn't matter. All that mattered is that I was there, and I was going to run all the way.

As we approached the first hill and started up the steep grade, my breathing became rapid, but I made it to the top with no problem. I was pacing myself because I knew the next hill was a long, steep grade. I ran up the second hill, and many more people ran past me. I kept telling myself that I could do this and I had only one more hill to go. The last hill was very steep and rocky, so I walked part of it. I had never been on the narrow trail with so many people at one time. I made it to the top, and one boy who looked to be about 11 years old started to pace me.

In my mind, I thought I cannot be beaten by a little boy. When we got to the top of the hill at the same time, I started running downhill as fast as I could. It was a rocky, steep decline with a lot of twists and turns, and the little boy paced me the entire way. When we got to the bottom of the hill, we were neck and neck as we hit the pavement and ran toward the high school.

We still had to get back to the school track and run around it one more time. I kept right up with him, even though my legs were feeling rubbery. We made it to the track running, and I just took off and ran as fast as I could around the track and past the finish line. There were people at the end handing out ribbons to the finishers. I grabbed my ribbon as I ran by. Tears flooded my eyes as I slowed my pace and walked around in a circle for a few seconds, catching my breath. People started congratulating me as I joined the other runners, who were congratulating each other.

People asked how long I had been running, and I told them three months. They were amazed that I was able to run the tough race when I'd just started running. I told them I'd also just survived colon cancer and recovered from a colon resection a few months earlier. They were astonished! Hearing their kind words made me feel even more proud of myself. For the first time in my life, I realized that I was amazing! Everyone said I should wait to see where I placed in the race. I stayed, even though I knew I didn't make the top groups. What I did not know was there were age groups, and I came in third in my age group. On this day, I became a runner.

Be determined to make exercise a joyful experience. Give exercise an important place in your life, because exercise can save it. Think of a time in your life when you achieved something big. Recreate the feeling in your mind. Visualize yourself enjoying every minute of your exercise program. If you're training for a race or some type of competition, visualize yourself finishing strong in your competition. Visualize success in your training and in everything you do in life. This is a very powerful way of training your mind as well as your body. Take that feeling and apply it to whatever type of exercise you do. Use your inner strength and positive feelings to get you to try new things and to find an exercise that you love.

Three months after I had colon resection, my dad had a major stroke. I was working at the school and the bank when my mom called to tell me. My son and I flew down to Los Angeles to be with my family and sit with my dad. He had already gone through brain surgery, had an aneurysm removed, and was sitting up and eating. He looked great, and he was talking to us and glad we were there. He wanted to go home, so the nurses sedated him, but they gave him too much medication, and his heart stopped while I was in the room.

I was rushed out by the nurse as the doctors started working to revive him. They were successful, but my dad suffered brain damage and didn't know who he was or what was going on. He developed water on the brain and was in a hospital and care facility for four months. My son and I drove five to six hours to Los Angeles from San Jose every weekend to visit him.

My dad physically recovered about four months later, but mentally, he was not the same. He couldn't live alone anymore, so he moved in with my mom and brothers. Over the next several years, he got dementia and then Alzheimer's, and the decline was severe. Alzheimer's is a terrible disease that takes its toll on the patient and the caregivers.

I thought about the strong man who was my father and how strict he was with me growing up. When I had surgery for cancer, he came to the hospital with my mom. They would walk me down the hallways of the hospital, pushing my IV pole and holding my arms as I took the painful steps I needed to recover. My dad always encouraged me to walk further each time, as he knew my determination, and he walked with me every morning and several times a day.

After I got out of the hospital, we walked around my neighborhood. My dad had to go back to Los Angeles to take care of his horses and work. My mom stayed an extra week to help me because I couldn't lift, bend, twist, or carry anything due to the large incision in my abdomen and the incisions reconnecting my colon. My mom found a group of ladies from the church to come and help me for the next several weeks. They went grocery shopping, did housework, and picked up my son from school.

When I was able to go to the store, I would ride with them. Their kindness was very much appreciated, and I promised to help others as soon as I was able to.

Events that knock you down in life may happen, but picking yourself up and charging forward is what matters. You cannot let anything keep you down. For me, being diagnosed and surviving a usually terminal disease at 36 shook my world. Some questions in my mind came up later, one being why did I get colon cancer? I thought there must be a higher purpose for me. Most people don't have any symptoms at the early stage I had. When life got back to normal, I began doing a lot of things that I never anticipated doing.

The first thing I wanted to do was get back to going to work, and working out at the gym. I waited the full eight weeks because I didn't want anything to tear anything or cause any problems during my recovery. When the doctor released me to normal activity, I worked into it slowly. If I had any discomfort or pain, I stopped.

Caution during recovery is vital to a good outcome. I felt God must want me to speak to people, to let them know young people get colon cancer and what the symptoms are. The fact that I conquered colon cancer made me a perfect spokesperson. I needed experience speaking in public, so I joined Toastmasters International to learn to speak to large groups. I joined the American Cancer Society to give speeches to cancer patients and give them hope for the future. I wrote public service announcements and spoke on television to reach a broader audience. I took every opportunity to speak about how I survived colon cancer and took questions afterward.

While I was out running in the hills, I would practice my speeches, sing songs, and thank God for my life and all the wonderful people in it. It was truly a life-changing time for me.

Running in the hills gave me the greatest feeling of joy, and I was happy to be alive.

After my colon cancer diagnosis and colon resection, things were going well. My workouts were going strong, my son started working out at the gym with me, and I started a new business as a traveling notary public, witnessing signatures on loan refinancing documents. This business gave me the ability to take care of my son and go to all his games and school events. I got a job at a television station as a videographer for the evening and late-night news.

Acting was something I had been doing part-time, and some of the commercials were shot locally and others were in San Francisco. A friend would pick me up and drive us to our location. She always told me if I brought broccoli and cauliflower, I would have to wait until we got there to eat it because it smelled up her car. We got a good laugh out of that, but bringing my own food was always a smart idea. We would end up on a TV or movie set for hours and sometimes late into the night, and everyone would come to me for food because they were starving and knew I always brought food.

When you don't eat enough food throughout the day, it's easy to become fatigued and sleepy due to low blood sugar. This was not a good condition to be in on the set when I was about to be on camera and needed to remember my lines. It was also not good to be on the road driving when hungry, tired, or not paying attention to the road or traffic. I saw many serious accidents while on the road, and I am always a very defensive and assertive driver, anticipating what is going to happen around me.

The businesses I started had me on the road all the time, driving from place to place, and I had a variety of experiences with distracted drivers. My first business was in Los Angeles, where the freeways were busy day and night and it seemed like no one ever slept. Every day, I saw people doing the dumbest things while driving. Men shaving their faces and pulling out nose hairs, and women putting on makeup. One man was reading a novel while driving in traffic on the 405 freeway, one of the busiest freeways in Los Angeles. On the same freeway, I saw a woman breastfeeding her baby while driving in traffic. There were people standing in the middle of the freeway looking at their car that broke down, or changing a tire in a lane of traffic. Many people have been hit by distracted drivers or someone texting or talking on their phone. It's still a distraction and should be avoided unless it's urgent, and any long conversations should be done while parked.

Early one Saturday morning, I had a loan document signing at a house 45 minutes away. I completed it and was on the way back on a street with a single lane going each way. There was a car coming toward me, and with no indication or blinker, the driver suddenly whipped in front of me. I slammed on the brakes and was honking the horn, but she kept coming. She hit the front of my car so hard that I thought she'd broken my back. My car spun around and she hit me again from the side.

When my car stopped spinning, I was in shock. The entire front of my car and my side door were smashed in. My body went into fight-or-flight mode, and I knew I had to get out of the car. I kicked the door open and got out and slowly stood up, unsure if my back was broken. When I was able to stand, I went to the window of the other car and started screaming at the woman. She rolled up the window but didn't get out.

Everyone in the neighborhood came running out of their houses and asked me if I was alright. They brought me food and water and a kitchen chair to sit on. They called the police, and the paramedics got there first. They asked the crowd of people if the person driving the car was deceased. The crowd spread out so I could be seen sitting in the chair, and I said, "I was driving the car."

The paramedics looked at my smashed-up car then back at me and said, "You walked out of that?" They said they'd never seen anyone get out of a wreck like that. They examined me and said an ambulance was on the way to take me to the hospital. I called my son and told him to come pick me up. We never had medical insurance; I always paid out of pocket for medical, dental, and vision. A few months prior, my son had to be taken to the hospital in an ambulance and I just paid off the $1,000 fee for the ride.

I told everyone I was fine. I just needed to go home and lay down. They insisted I go to the hospital. They said I was in shock and couldn't feel the extent of my injuries. Against the professional judgment of the paramedics, I went home with my son. In the morning, I woke up and couldn't move. My son had to drive me to the hospital. The fact that I was able to withstand the impact without any broken bones was a testament to how strong I was, and how exercise and healthy eating had made me strong enough to survive the impact of a big vehicle traveling 35 miles per hour that hit me head-on and again from the side.

The ER doctor said I was very lucky to survive such a serious accident. He did a lot of x-rays and then showed me that I had no broken bones but should have been seen right after the accident. He said I had sprains and strains on my spine and that it would take a few months to recover. I told him there was no way I could take time off. I'd just started a new company and didn't have medical insurance or sick days, and I was a single parent. He said I had no choice. I had to rest and recover.

A few days later, I still couldn't move. Everything hurt, but I wanted to go to my Toastmasters meeting, and I needed my son to drive me. One of the members was a chiropractor who said he would treat me for free and had a good attorney for me to use. The next day, I saw the chiropractor and the attorney, but sitting in the office, I was in terrible pain. The attorney had me sign the paperwork so he could get started on my case, and he said he'd make sure my chiropractor was covered for as many visits as I needed to get better.

My son drove me home, and I lay on the couch wondering what I could do to get better faster. This was not like my colon resection because I really didn't know what was wrong with me or how long it would take. The chiropractor wanted me to come to his office every day and get adjustments and traction, which was very painful. I still couldn't sit or drive, and the pain was severe. The attorney told me I could go to a medical doctor to get another evaluation.

After weeks of being off work and in severe pain, I went to a sports orthopedist. He said my injuries were severe and I was lucky to be alive. He said he could give me an injection of steroids to help ease the pain, but I still needed to stay off work and let my body heal. He had me lay on a table, and I watched him load a huge needle with medication. He stuck the giant needle into my tailbone, and I almost jumped off the table. It seemed like it took 10 minutes for him to finish. The doctor said I would feel better in a few days, but I still had to stay off work and exercise for six to eight weeks. Why did I get the shot if I had to stay off everything? It did make me feel better, thought, and he said I could walk if it didn't make the pain worse. I would have to return in a week to check my progress. If I was still in a lot of pain, he would do more x-rays. This was enough pain relief after two days for me to start walking at the track near my home.

Steroid injections can be very helpful to minimize pain from an injury or car accident. I am not a doctor, but from my experience, a steroid shot can be helpful. The shot can greatly reduce pain, but that doesn't mean you should return to normal activity. The doctor may recommend rest for a few days after the injection or in some cases, walking for exercise. Follow the instructions of the doctor and don't rush back to activity. I had a lot of physical, chiropractic, and acupuncture therapy after my accident, and I didn't return to vigorous activity until the doctor said it was okay. Swimming was the first activity I was able to do because it didn't put stress on my injuries. It took time before I was able to start swimming, and I followed the doctor's instructions. Most doctors will not recommend alternative treatments, but I feel they helped me. Life is not always smooth sailing, but having colon cancer, a colon resection, and a severe car accident three years later was a lot to deal with. My car was a total loss, but it could be replaced.

My recommendation when you have an injury, especially a car accident, is to see a doctor for an evaluation. It's difficult to know how bad you're hurt when you're in a car accident because the body starts pumping adrenaline and endorphins to increase physical alertness and elevate mood. This is how your body protects itself, also known as acute stress response. This is the fight-or-flight response. The adrenaline response enabled me to kick my smashed door open. The endorphins, also the hormone released during exercise that makes you feel good, can make it difficult to know how badly you are hurt. There are instances when people can lift a car to save someone pinned underneath. In my case, I kicked my way out of my car and stood up, making me think my injuries were not serious.

It's hard to take time off when you're used to working out every day, but there are times when it's necessary. If you get injured, it's important to seek medical attention. If your doctor gives you permission to walk or lift weights, then you can continue with a modified workout until you heal. If the doctor tells you to rest, it's best to rest. It doesn't do any good to try to work through an injury.

I have had a few injuries that required time off to heal. When I was a runner, I got an Achilles tendon injury. I wanted to keep running, but it was too painful. I went to the trail in the hills and started walking and stretching. There was another runner who was walking behind a group of runners. I started talking to him, and he told me he was with the running group but had an injury and had to walk, so we walked together each morning until we eventually were able to run again. I got to meet all the people in the running club and made new friends. They became a support system of motivated people helping each other keep going no matter what. It's smart to let your body heal and repair, which is very important to your long-term recovery. I was able to go from walking to swimming and then back to running.

There are many people who have had a serious injury or illness and are unable to exercise. This may be temporary, or they may be disabled for life. I can tell you every time I've had an injury, surgery, or am hurting, I see someone who's in worse shape. Someone who is missing an arm or a leg or is in a wheelchair, and I think, *I have nothing to be feeling down about. I have everything I need to overcome anything that comes my way!* If you find yourself unable to do something that you love, find something motivating like watching people who have recovered from injury or lost a limb and are still able to find activities they can do. Then ask yourself what your limitation is. I think you'll see the only thing holding you back are the thoughts in your head.

After an injury, your movement may be limited depending on the injury, but find something that you can do. I've seen tennis players with leg or ankle injuries sitting in a chair and hitting the tennis ball. If you have an injury to your lower body, do upper-body exercises. If the injury is to your upper body, do leg exercises and cardiovascular exercises. Clear any exercise program with your doctor if you're starting something new or are under a doctor's care. A chiropractor is a good resource when it comes to knowing what you should and should not do after an injury. If something is causing you pain, don't keep doing it. Pushing through pain will delay your recovery and could cause serious damage or make the injury worse. Make sure if you're not getting better to see a chiropractor or a doctor. Seek many opinions and alternative therapy such as Pilates, yoga, chiropractic care, and acupuncture. The strength you're building every day at the gym can save your life, and you can add that to the list of reasons you should lift weights and do strength training and cardiovascular exercise. The benefits of exercise are countless and make it the best thing you can do for your body.

Life's challenges
After taking acting classes, I got headshots taken and started going on auditions for television and movie gigs. I ended up getting a lot of jobs doing commercials and TV shows such as *Nash Bridges*, and I was in the movie *Patch Adams*. I got to meet Robin Williams and spent a lot of time talking with him. I also got to meet the real Patch Adams, who was on the set every day. The makeup ladies on the set were having fun with Patch Adams wearing makeup. He posed for a photo with me while I was made up for my part in the movie. I still have that picture on my desk. This just goes to prove that when you put your mind to something, great things happen. I focused on being successful in television, movies, and commercials, and that is exactly what happened. It was great fun, and I loved every minute of it.

Not knowing what to do or where to start can sometimes stop people from doing things. Just go out and do something. It doesn't matter what it is, as long as you're moving your body and having fun. Some people will say the best part of working out is when they're done. They really love it, or they wouldn't be there. Don't let the fear of being different or not being as fit as someone else stop you from joining in. I jumped into acting with both feet and I had a lot of fun and got to meet a lot of famous people and see myself on television and in films at the theater. I did a lot of great things by becoming a spokesperson for the America Cancer Society. I also used my acting experience to make public service announcements to let people know that young people get colon cancer. It's not just a disease old people get. I was the youngest person they had ever met who had colon cancer at 36. These days, colon cancer is being seen in young people and even in children. Know the signs and know your family history.

When I worked as a notary public, I also acted and did some videography work. I had already done several commercials and television shows when I got a gig to do a commercial in San Francisco. While I was doing cardiovascular exercise, I would run my lines. This was a perfect time for me to rehearse a speech and lines for auditions and upcoming commercials and television shows.

One day, I got a call from my agent telling me I had a national commercial that would be filmed in two days. He sent me the lines, and I rehearsed many times so I would be prepared. When I went to bed that night, I knew all my lines and had my clothes set out so I could get up early and be ready to go. At 3:00 a.m., the phone rang. I answered, and it was my mom. She was crying as she told me my dad had died. He got up to go to the bathroom, fell, and didn't get up. It must have been a heart attack.

My heart sank in my chest. She asked how soon I could fly down with my son. She knew I had a commercial that day, in just a few hours. I said, "I know Dad would want me to do my commercial. We'll fly down on an evening flight." One of the hardest things I ever had to do was drive to the location and shoot a commercial as if nothing was wrong. Before I got to the location, I pulled over and prayed for God to give me the strength to get through this without breaking down. I wiped the tears from my eyes and fixed my makeup and put a smile on my face and drove to my location and did the commercial.

We never know what is going to happen in life. There are always peaks and valleys, highs and lows. Some say we must prepare for the worst and hope for the best. I say prepare for the best and always give 100% at whatever you do. My dad would always say, "Go on with it!" That is what I did.

When one door closes, another one opens. I just lost my dad, and a few days later I met Jerry Dwyer, who would end up being my future husband. Sadly, my dad passed away before he got to meet Jerry, but I know he is looking down from heaven saying, "Go on with it!"

Don't let life get you down or defeat you. It's all part of the journey. Have as many positive people in your life and activities in your life as possible, and everything will work out. Never stop believing that.

Putting your health as your number-one priority is extremely important. If you don't take good care of yourself, you can't take care of anyone else. When your health is great, you feel great, look great, and can help other people. Many diseases can be avoided by taking care of yourself from an early age, but it's never too late to start. Exercise and maintaining a healthy weight and diet can lower cholesterol and blood pressure, and defeat type 2 diabetes and many cancers.

An aneurysm is a dilation in the wall of an artery supplying blood to a specific area. It causes pain, dizziness, nausea, vomiting, rapid heart rate, low blood pressure, and shock. Cholesterol can combine with fat, calcium, and other substances in the blood to form plaque. When plaque builds up in the arteries, it causes them to narrow. An aneurysm can be prevented by maintaining a healthy weight, eating healthy foods, and exercising on a regular basis. Other things to avoid are smoking and weight gain. Alcohol should be avoided or limited. The blood flow to major organs becomes limited and causes several health issues, including blood clots. A blood clot can lead to heart attack and death. This is another reason to eat healthily and exercise daily. Do not wait until you have a serious condition to begin taking care of yourself.

Meeting Jerry

While running at Rancho San Antonio, I would pray for a wonderful man to come into my life. I prayed for a man who was smart, educated, handsome, loving, active, with a good sense of humor, and who would love me unconditionally. I met my future husband, Jerry Dwyer, 30 days after praying at the top of the hill. He is all the things I prayed for and so much more. We started working out together and going on hikes and running those same hills. Some of the best ideas always came to me when I was running. Being outside with nature gets your blood flowing and makes you feel alive. Take advantage of being outside in nature as much as possible. Even if you're just going for a walk, it's a fabulous way to start your day and an effective way to burn calories.

Jerry had torn his anterior cruciate ligament (ACL) when we first met. He couldn't run, but he would go to Rancho San Antonio with me and walk the flat trails while I ran in the hills. We would meet on the low trail and walk back to the parking lot. The fact that he couldn't run didn't stop me from asking him to come with me and from him accepting my offer. This was his exercise while he awaited approval for his surgery. He was a major in the U.S. Army and worked at Santa Clara University and Stanford University teaching military science. We met by chance and knew early in our relationship that we were meant to be together.

Jerry always wanted to learn how to eat healthier. Being an army aviator kept him on the go during the early part of his career. He had flown many years prior to meeting me and was sent to California for a few years. He never wore a uniform, so I didn't feel like he was really in the Army until the day he was taking the cadets on a training exercise and he was in his uniform. He looked so handsome! I realized at that point he was really in the Army. It was the first time we were apart, and I really missed him.

We did everything together. One difference was that he went to the gym at the university during lunch, and I went to the gym in the early morning before work. I owned my own business, so I could make my own hours to a certain degree, but I did have to start around eight o'clock. I asked Jerry to join my gym so we could work out together, and we've been working out together in the mornings ever since.

When to modify your exercise
Once you get in the habit of exercising, it'll make you feel so good that you'll want to keep moving no matter what is happening. This is when you know you're unstoppable and can handle anything. It's a feeling that drives you to get up early and exercise hard. Making a positive change motivates you to do things that you never thought were possible. It's an amazing feeling.

Modify your exercise if you're not feeling well or if you're tired. If you're feeling exhausted or sick, take the day off from exercise.

You can go for a walk or do a yoga DVD or find an exercise show or just do some stretching at home. Yoga is beneficial for the immune system and for calming the mind and body. Don't push yourself when you have the flu or any virus, as this may prolong your illness. One or two days off from the gym will not hurt you. Pushing yourself or exercising when you're sick is not a good idea and may hurt you.

There may be days when you just feel bored or tired with your exercise routine or need a change of pace. Try taking a class at the gym or going on a run or a walk with a friend. Make plans to meet with a friend or go out to lunch after your workout. Sometimes, you need a little variation to your exercise or daily routine to put the life back into your exercise program.

There will be times when you're unable to work out. The most important thing to do is to maintain a healthy eating plan. You won't need to eat as many calories as you do when you're running or working out hard. Cut out some of the extra calories by eating smaller portions. Do not diet at this time, because your body still needs calories to keep running strong. Stay away from all junk and empty-calorie foods and concentrate on organic fruits and vegetables and lean protein. By doing this, you can maintain your fitness and keep your weight in check.

Don't drink alcohol while you're in recovery from an injury or when you're taking medication or antibiotics. Alcohol will kill your gains faster than anything else. Alcohol causes weight gain due to extra calories and slows your metabolism. When your body is trying to heal, it's important to give it the nutrients it needs. Staying on my healthy eating plan will ensure that you're giving your body what it needs to heal.

Eat a lot of fruit because it has vitamin C, fiber, and phytochemicals along with additional vitamins your body needs to get and stay healthy. Eat lean protein to maintain your muscle and lots of vegetables for vitamins and fiber.

Surgery, alternatives, and therapy

I am not a doctor so I cannot give you medical advice, but I have been a patient several times in my life. The most important thing to know about surgery is whether it is absolutely necessary and if there are alternative treatments to try first. If you have a sore knee or shoulder, massage, acupuncture, or physical therapy should be tried first, unless you have broken bones or a condition that requires surgery. If surgery is recommended, become well informed and ask the doctor every question about the surgery, what your limitations are after the surgery, and what type of exercise you'll be able to do during the recovery.

Before agreeing to a surgery of any form, consider less invasive alternatives like cardiovascular exercise, weightlifting, stretching, and Pilates. Find a Pilates instructor who knows how to work with people who have back pain or whatever physical problem you have. Yoga is good for stretching and deep breathing and relaxation. Yoga, Pilates, and strength training along with cardiovascular exercises such as an elliptical trainer, spinning bike, biking outside, running, or walking will all get you in shape as long as your surgeon is okay with doing them before and after surgery. Find out what you will not be able to do if you have an elective surgery such as back surgery, knee or hip surgery, or cervical surgery. Being restricted for the rest of your life may make the surgery less appealing.

Exercise can prevent the need for surgery, and in many cases may make it unnecessary. Most spine surgeries don't need to be done immediately, according to what I was told by a doctor who was honest about spine surgery to reduce pain. In fact, many people who undergo spine surgery end up with more pain or describe it as a different type of pain, some of which can be debilitating.

If you're having back pain or leg pain and a doctor tells you back surgery will eliminate it, get a second and third opinion. The doctor I trusted most told me that it is very difficult to treat back pain and that he turns down many surgeries because of the poor outcome. If surgery is mandatory due to the severity of an injury, that may be a different story. Each case has to be evaluated, but look for alternatives whenever possible. Use exercise, physical therapy, chiropractic, acupuncture, Pilates, and yoga as alternatives. When the pain is flared up, rest or do something gentle on the body like walking or Pilates. Do whatever you can to avoid any type of spine surgery. It's a nightmare surgery and recovery, does little to cure your back pain, and typically creates a new set of problems.

Pilates
Pilates is one of the greatest forms of exercise I have found to keep my body strong and maintain my health. Joseph Pilates invented the first reformer as a way to treat and rehabilitate soldiers injured in World War I. The success of this technique was so great that it continues to be applied the way it was originally intended, and since that time it has become a popular fitness technique. Pilates focuses on core strength, comprising movements that enhance balance, mobility, flexibility, core strength, and breathing that relaxes and settles the body. Pilates helps enhance good feelings. It's very important to maintain core strength to support your entire body. This is one of the ways I have found that improves my ability to function on many levels. My first Pilates class was on a DVD, and I used it three times a week to do Pilates on a mat at home.

When looking for a Pilates instructor, I recommend finding

someone who pays close attention to make sure you're using the correct form and getting the core muscles activated. I went to several instructors before I found the right one: Kristina. Pilates instructors are in abundance, but finding one who watches every move using knowledge and intuition is hard to find. The best instructors have experience with a variety of clients and know about back problems, so the movements you do are good for your body.

Kristina taught me how to use my core strength and how to avoid flaring up my sciatic nerve while I was exercising. She also taught me how to recognize things that may not be the best for my body and how to relieve the pain if it flared up. She is very intuitive and a wonderful instructor. Not all instructors have her knowledge and intuition. Every time I go to Hermosa Beach, I get on her schedule and work with her while I am in town. She helped me get my small muscles to work without the large muscles taking over.

My exercise

The morning routine is going to the gym to do an hour of cardiovascular exercise on the elliptical or spinning bike, then lifting weights for 30 minutes doing two body parts, and ending with core exercise. Each day, I do two different body parts: the first day, back and triceps; the next day, chest and biceps; the third day, legs and shoulders. Then repeat.

During the week, I get up at 3:00 a.m., drink a whole glass of water, eat a piece of toast, and head for the gym. My gym is open 24 hours a day, so I can work out any time I want, but mornings work best for me because there is nothing I need to do at 4:00 a.m. I ride the stationary bike or use the elliptical trainer for an hour, then lift weights for 30 minutes and do 10 minutes of core exercises.

Jerry and I work out together every morning. We get home by 6:00 a.m. and have a bowl of oatmeal with protein powder and almond milk mixed in, with fresh berries, slivered almonds, and pumpkin seeds on top. On Sunday, I make a big pot of oatmeal, which only takes a few minutes to heat up and serve for breakfast throughout the week. This is a helpful time saver. When I'm at the gym, I listen to music on my iPod because I don't want the interruptions that come from using my phone. My workout has my undivided attention. Doing interval training, such as pedaling fast for three minutes then slow for 30 seconds then back to fast pace, burns a lot of calories.

On the weekends, we get up at 4:00 a.m., sometimes 5:00 a.m., and ride our spinning bikes at home while we watch a concert or music show on the DVR with a fast energetic beat. I can burn 500 to 600 calories while listening to music or watching *Dancing with the Stars*, alternating speeds and adjusting the tension for a lot of variety and an enjoyable workout. After our ride, we go lift weights at the gym. If time is limited, we can lift weights and use exercise bands at home. There is always a way to fit some type of workout into our mornings. Anyone starting an exercise program for the first time, or anyone with health issues, should consult their doctor prior to beginning an exercise program.

When I travel, I have a gym close by so I can continue to work out each day that's not a travel day. I love to go back to California where I grew up and visit my family. My husband has business there, so we visit every few months. We always go to my favorite restaurant, The Spot, which is a vegetarian restaurant with many meal options, and Good Stuff by the beach. Both have food made with healthy ingredients and no artificial ingredients. Captain Kidd's Fish Market in Redondo Beach has the best fresh fish. We buy fish every day and cook it at the hotel.

I'm always doing whatever I can to stay healthy, whether at home or traveling. Going to the gym in the morning, taking walks on the beach, riding bikes, and lying in the sun. I have a trainer, Kate, who I work with when she's available. She teaches exercises in a supportive, positive way and is fun to work with.

I tried to find Pilates instructors where I live but didn't find anyone who was right for me. I decided to buy a Pilates Reformer for my house and work on my own doing the routines Kristina taught me. I can learn routines from Kristina and practice them when I get back home. I use them three or four times a week when I'm at home.

Pilates can be done on a floor mat with a wide variety of movements that all focus on the core to improve stability. The Pilates Reformer is a table that has springs, ropes, and pulleys, which improve strength, particularly in the core, back, glutes, and thighs, along with flexibility and balance, coordination posture, and body alignment. There are a wide variety of movements that can be done standing, sitting, and lying down. There is also a table called the Reformer Cadillac or Trapeze Table, and there are a variety of movements that can be done from a suspended position using a series of springs, pulleys, a trapeze, and a push-through bar. I have the Studio Reformer with Tower, which converts to a Cadillac Reformer and enables work on multiple platforms, and from both sides.

Breathing

It sounds simple because breathing happens automatically and you don't have to remind yourself to breathe. Knowing how to breathe is what you need to know. Every second of life, our hearts are pumping blood and our lungs are filled up with air when we inhale and push out air when we exhale. The definition of breathing is the process of moving air in and out of the lungs to facilitate gas exchange with the internal environment, mostly to flush out carbon dioxide and bring in oxygen. This is an automatic process that is part of bodily function that goes on inside the body and keeps us alive.

What happens to our breathing when we're under stress is something that we need to be aware of. Stress changes the pattern of breathing from normal diaphragm breathing to small, shallow breaths, using the shoulders rather than the diaphragm to move air in and out of the lungs. Breathing becomes faster to distribute oxygen-rich blood to your body. Those who already have breathing problems will find it even harder to breathe under stress. Learning deep breathing techniques will help lower your heart rate and make you feel relaxed. Rapid breathing disrupts the balance of gases in the body. The heart pumps faster, and stress can increase inflammation in the body, which in turn is linked to factors that can cause heart problems such as high blood pressure and lower "good" HDL cholesterol.

Deep breathing combats anxiety and stimulates the parasympathetic nervous system, which makes you feel more relaxed. The parasympathetic nervous system is the opposite of the fight-or-flight term of action for the sympathetic nervous system. Instead of getting you ready for the action response, deep breathing gets you to relax. Deep breaths decrease your blood pressure, dilate your pupils, and slow your heart rate, which lowers the arousal response in the process. When you take deep breaths in through the nose and out through the mouth and make the out-breath longer, it helps to bring about relaxation and slows down the heart rate. A rapid heart rate can keep you from getting a good night's sleep. Longer breathing stimulates this response.

The difference is that deep diaphragmatic breathing occurs

when your diaphragm moves down and pushes your stomach out as you take a breath, rather than shallower lung breathing. Shallow breathing raises blood pressure and brings about anxiety in the mind and body. The way to do this is to breathe in for seven counts and out for 11 counts. Continue this type of breathing until you notice a calming effect.

Be aware of your breathing and how your diaphragm moves up and down, and let your muscles relax. If you can do this lying down, let your ribs melt into the back of your body. Exhale all the air completely and have the out-breath be longer than the in-breath for the most relaxing benefit. Breathing stimulates the lymphatic system, which detoxifies the body and helps remove toxins from the body. Deep breathing lowers blood pressure, improves digestion, and helps support correct posture. Anytime you're feeling anxious, take 10 minutes to do some deep, relaxing breathing exercises.

One effective way to fall asleep is to listen to guided meditation, which uses breathing and visualization to help you relax and fall asleep. There are many places to find relaxation, sleep music, or guided imagery. They can be found on CDs or online, and there are apps that you can download, which are helpful also.

Massage relieves stress and tight muscles through a sports deep-tissue massage or a Swedish massage. One of my massage therapists in California is Jelica, who works on the tight areas of my body to relieve pain and improve circulation. Another one of my massage therapists from California, Dann, does a type of releasing massage where he works into a tight area and has me breathe and release the area. I have to work during this type of massage with my breathing and relaxing the muscles. Dann tells me to notice where I'm holding or resisting, and to let the muscle go and release it. This has been one of the most relaxing types of massage I have found. I get on his schedule whenever I'm in California.

Acupuncture is a form of alternative medicine in which thin needles are placed in various areas of the body to increase blood flow and relieve pain while releasing stress in the body. Acupuncture stimulates the central nervous system by releasing chemicals into the muscles, spinal cord, and brain, which may stimulate the body's natural healing. I find it to be very relaxing and reduces pain.

Jerry's surgery

Jerry had to have surgery to repair his completely torn ACL just a few months after we met. The surgeon was at Stanford University in Palo Alto, close to the hills where we ran. The surgery went smoothly, but Jerry was on crutches with a heavy-duty brace that had adjustments on the angle for his knee. The ACL can't repair itself and they needed to take a tendon from his knee to do the repair. They had him walking on the crutches a few hours after surgery, showing him how to use them to walk and get up the stairs. He would start physical therapy several weeks later.

We really got to know each other very well over this time. He needed me to help him in and out of bed and on and off the toilet. I remembered how much pain I was in after my colon resection and how much help I needed. This was a painful process. Jerry had never had surgery or taken pain medication. He was determined not to take anything, but the next day, the pain got so bad he took one pill at bedtime and slept for eight hours. When he woke up, he said, "Never give me those again." He used the Motrin for the next few days, and then it was tolerable.

In between my work, I went to make his meals and help him get around. I also gave him core exercises that he could do while on the floor with his leg propped up on the coffee table. Then I had to run back to my house and take care of my son. He was almost 21, so I didn't need to do much, but I made his food and got some work done. I picked up my documents for work the next day and then went back to take care of Jerry.

I nursed Jerry through the recovery and helped him with everything. We did core exercises and some Pilates to strengthen his body without using his leg. His physical therapist was shocked by how strong and ahead of the recovery process Jerry was. He was where most patients were after weeks of physical therapy. I knew it was the healthy eating and exercise, and Jerry and his therapist were both convinced. The therapist had to figure out new exercises for Jerry to do because everything he usually gave ACL patients was too easy. This is just another example of how exercise and healthy eating speed up healing.

Through Jerry's recovery from ACL surgery, I got to know his parents very well. They lived in Arizona since Jerry was a young boy, and before that, his dad was an aviator in the U.S. Air Force. Ann and Jerry Sr. were so optimistic about everything. They always asked if we needed anything and were only concerned with how we were doing. They thanked me for taking care of Jr., which is what they called him. During one of our phone calls, his mother casually mentioned having her gallbladder taken out as if it was no big deal. I was surprised and concerned about her, but she said she was fine. The next week, she said she had to get one of her kidneys removed, and I was really worried she might have cancer.

I asked Jerry, and he said they never wanted to worry the kids (he had two sisters and a brother), so they kept everything to themselves. The next time I talked to her, she was going to the doctor again, and I asked if they said she may have cancer. She told me the doctors said they thought they got it all and she was fine.

This was very scary to me, and I told Jerry he should call and ask his mom. We both listened as she downplayed the diagnosis and said she was fine.

They don't take out organs one after another unless cancer had spread. Jerry talked to his dad, and he confirmed she had cancer. They were only worried about Jerry Jr. and said she would be fine and the doctors were taking good care of her. We planned to visit them in Arizona as soon as Jerry recovered. We were able to visit his parents several times, and everything seemed fine, but regardless of the positive attitude and optimism, I knew it was very serious.

Every visit was the same, where everything was going great and his parents wanted to make sure we were doing well. His dad would always say, "Take time to put your feet up and relax" and "Always look to the future and don't worry about anything."

At one point, Jerry's mom mentioned the doctor finding a spot on her liver. I knew the cancer was very serious and had spread. We stayed in a hotel by his parents' house and went to the gym in the morning. After breakfast, we went to visit them. There was never a time when they were downbeat. Mom always said she felt the medication was working well and dad talked finances and aviation with Jr. as they had his whole life.

9/11

Three years after we met, Jerry was given command of a Chinook helicopter unit at Fort Hood, Texas. He was ecstatic to be going back to flying, and I was terrified because it meant he was going to war in Iraq or Afghanistan. I had only been to Texas one time previously and was unfamiliar with the weather and the state. This was a time to be strong, and it was a two-year command and then we thought we would be back in California.

We drove across the country so I could bring Jerry to flight training on the Chinook helicopter at Fort Rucker in Enterprise, Alabama. On the drive, we stopped at hotels near the healthiest restaurants we could find. We got up in the mornings to run and had breakfast before hitting the road again. I had never been on a cross-country drive. We stopped to visit his parents and then continued to Alabama.

I was a vegetarian, and I found it was harder to find food once we got past Arizona. The hotel and motels were smaller, and the accommodations were less than I normally encountered. We learned a lot about each other on that drive, and I realized how big this country is and how different every state is. Finding steamed vegetables, decent salads, chicken breasts, or fish without breading or being fried became difficult. I decided to pick up things from the grocery store to make sandwiches so we wouldn't have to stop for lunch. For breakfast, there were no scrambled egg whites, so I just ordered hard-boiled eggs and took the yolk out. I bought Ezekiel Bread from the store for my breakfast and got rice cakes and trail mix to snack on.

When we arrived in Alabama, I was shocked that no restaurants were open because it was Sunday. We were able to find one place that was open and had fish, but the only vegetable was fried okra. I was not in California anymore. I couldn't wait to fly back home and get back to the gym and healthy food, but I did learn that no matter where I was, I could find a place to run and create my own healthy meals.

Two months after I dropped Jerry off at Fort Rucker, he came home for what was our last few days in California. We packed everything we needed for the drive: toiletries, clean clothes, gym clothes, and shoes. Jerry didn't have time to go through his boxes in the garage that had piled up from every move he'd since he joined the Army. The movers came and packed up everything, including our bed, and took it to Texas to store until we found a place to live.

The move to Fort Hood

We always take our gym clothes and running gear when we travel so we can work out and or take a run. Planning to work out every day makes it easier to accomplish. It's too easy to put it off. The plan is to always work out wherever we go, and we do even if it's raining. We got stuck in the middle of nowhere a few times and started running, and the rain started coming down in sheets. I never saw it rain so hard. We were soaked by the time we got back to the hotel.

During this move, we visited Arizona and Jerry's parents, who were optimistic as always, but his mom was not doing well. It took us three drives from California to Texas, and every time, we stopped to see his mom. I was excited to show her my engagement ring. By the time we got there, she was in the hospital. She was as positive as always and didn't want to bother the nurses over the little pain she had in her side. I called the nurse and asked if she could make her more comfortable. We had to leave the next day for Jerry to report in for duty at Fort Hood. His dad had given us his Saturn Vue to use during our move, and we left our red Mustang convertible at his parents' house.

We had to spend a month in a hotel while we looked for a house to rent. The microwave was the only thing I had to cook with, so I made scrambled eggs, vegetables, potatoes, Amy's Burritos, and sandwiches for lunch. Dinner was usually salad, vegetables, and some type of protein, either tofu or fish.

Every day, we went out for a run and then Jerry went to work, and I looked for a house to rent. While I was driving around, I found markets that had different types of frozen organic meals to make for dinner, and packaged salads. There were many houses for sale, but not many for rent. There were no trees in the areas near Fort Hood, so we looked for houses in the town of Belton. After weeks of looking, we found a place in Morgan's Point Resort, which was a wildlife preserve with lots of deer and trees. The trees were short, but it was the only place in the area with trees. There was a three-bedroom house for rent by the owners, who'd just moved out to build a bigger house. It was perfect and already decorated with drapes and nice fixtures. Neither of us was good at decorating, which made this the perfect place for us. We signed the papers and called the movers to bring our belongings to our new house.

The next morning, we packed up everything from the hotel and moved into our new home for the next two years. The movers were going to bring everything over that afternoon. We sat on the floor of our empty house, waiting for the movers. The phone company had already come to put the phone line in, and we got the television line ready along with internet service. As we sat inside our empty home waiting for the truck to bring our things, the phone rang. Jerry answered it, and within a minute his expression went from happy to sad. I knew that meant his mom had passed away. We both started to cry. We sat there on the floor of our empty new rental home, crying in each other's arms.

The way of the military is much different than anything I had experienced. My dad was in the Navy long before I was born. My uncle was in the Air Force, but I was in school and taking care of my brothers at the time. I wasn't sure what we were going to do. Jerry said if we didn't wait for the furniture to be delivered, it could take weeks to get back on the schedule, and we didn't have any clothes, suitcases, or anything. As we waited for the movers to arrive, we got calls from his sister, and I called my mom to let her know Jerry's mom had passed away.

It seemed like an eternity before the movers arrived. We didn't really know what we were doing. We told them to put the boxes marked for the kitchen into the kitchen, the boxes with clothes into the bedroom, and to set up the furniture. We had to go through all of the boxes of clothes to find something to wear to the funeral. We unloaded just what we needed and left the rest in the boxes and went to sleep.

The next morning, we flew to Arizona for the funeral. It was very difficult to walk into the mortuary. In the military, there's a lot of death, but nothing like the death of a parent, especially someone as special as Jerry's mom. We didn't want to view the body, but his sisters led us into the viewing area and we both broke down emotionally and had to leave. We wanted to remember his mother alive, smiling, and happy, as she had been throughout her life and to her very last breath.

The funeral service was traditional, with family members in attendance who came from different states. I met the extended family for the first time, and they were all lovely. We all went to a restaurant and talked and ate in celebration of a life now passed. After we were done, we went back to the family home with Jerry's dad, brother, and sisters. We visited with his family for a long time. Our Mustang was still at dad's house, so we drove it back to the hotel.

Jerry had to return to Fort Hood to his position as commander of the Chinook unit he was training to deploy to Afghanistan. It felt strange to be leaving so soon without a proper grieving period. But this was the military, and most of his family had been in the military, including one of his sisters, so they knew the protocol.

We drove to the house the next morning to drop off the car

and get a ride to the airport. We visited with the family and looked at old photos. Jerry showed me his childhood bedroom with all the airplane models hanging from the ceiling just the way he left it when he went to college.

Getting on a plane was the last thing we wanted to do. We needed to decompress, and the best way to do that was to get into the Mustang, put the top down, and drive back to Texas. We canceled our flight and jumped into the convertible and took off.

The plan was to drive to Fredericksburg, Texas, to spend the night and drive the rest of the way home the next morning. When we arrived in town, everything was packed with motorcycles and people having a big celebration. We got some gas and kept going. We got home late that night and slept a few hours. Then we got up, put on our running gear, and went for a run. We went to a little breakfast restaurant and ate, then went back home to shower. He got dressed in his battle gear and I put on my unpacking clothes. He went to Fort Hood and I started unpacking boxes and organizing our new life in Texas.

Organize your life

Life is filled with many events that we don't anticipate, and some that we know are going to happen. Regardless of what is going on in life, it's important to be organized. The amount of stuff collected over the years can become overwhelming. Everything comes with accessories like chargers, equipment, books, paper, parts, and pieces. When added to what you already have, these things can become clutter if you're not organized. Clutter can cause you to feel overwhelmed and make it difficult to concentrate. Some people get so distracted by clutter that they can't get anything done. For those people, controlling the clutter is essential to their health.

Anything that comes into your home should have a place to go like a cabinet, drawer, hanging file, or hanger. When you don't have a place to put things and just put them on the countertop, clutter starts to pile up. When you aren't organized, the mind can't focus as well, making it very difficult to be productive. Being organized is the best way to keep your home, office, and car from looking like a big mess.

Where do you start when your house is a cluttered mess and your workplace is disorderly? Take one drawer, closet, or room at a time and clean it out. Anything that you aren't using, give to a second-hand store or any place that'll take it off your hands. If you have clothes that you haven't worn in the past year, give them away. If the clothes are worn out, throw them away. Any parts and pieces that are incomplete or that you don't use anymore, throw them away. Get rid of everything that's holding you back from being organized and productive. Store things that are significant but not used in daily life, and donate things that are in good shape but not essential to your success. File papers that you need to reference in hanging files and use organizers to put the things you use daily in spaces where you can access them easily. Being organized creates more time for things that are fun and makes life a wonderful experience.

A home office can be a productive place to work when you don't have an office to work out of, but it can also be very distracting. The phone rings for non-business calls, people are coming in and out, daily household chores need to be done, and if you're not organized and disciplined, you can get distracted. This is where being organized will help you focus on work and you can divide your time between work and housework.

Schedule your time so you can fit exercise in before or after work, and make sure that you schedule time for a healthy lunch. Keep things in your refrigerator that are cooked and chopped to speed up the time it takes to make your meals. Working from home, especially if you have your own business, can be very difficult. The television is there as a distraction, and mindless eating can lead to weight gain. This is another time when organization and scheduling are key to success.

Make sure you keep to a schedule as much as possible. Wake up at the same time every day and work out. Take a shower, get dressed, and start work. Stop for a quick mid-morning snack and then work until lunch. After eating, go right back to work and keep working until it's time for a mid-afternoon snack. Continue working until it's time to stop for the day. Then make dinner and relax.

The other things that you need to do can be put in the appropriate places in your day. Don't turn on the television or anything that will distract you from getting your work done during the day. Meals can be eaten at the same time every day, which makes it easy to stick with a healthy meal and snack because they can be prepared in advance. If you go to the office, take your food with you, and keep to your schedule there. Have a time for e-mails and text messages that doesn't distract from your core job. Social media and emails come in all day long ,which takes the focus off work. Set aside time to deal with these without interfering with your work.

Flexibility

Life is full of schedules for everything from work, school, activities, and social events to unscheduled, unplanned events, car accidents, illness, hospitalization, and death. Nothing is certain but death and taxes. Many of us have seen this in our own lives and wonder why these things happen and what we can count on. The questions are infinite, and the answers are also. The truth of being successful in life is that you have to be ready for everything life throws your way. The key is to be flexible. Is flexibility just a figment of our imagination, or is it attainable? Flexible people adapt quickly to new situations, and they stay in control. Being able to think on your feet is something that you need to do in every situation in life. When a fastball comes out of left field, be flexible.

Life doesn't stop
In life, we all go through difficult times, but not everyone processes things in the same way. Everything happens so fast in the military. When Jerry's mom passed away, we were sad to lose her. We were bowled over by the news because she kept telling us the medicine and chemotherapy were working. She was a wonderful, positive person throughout her life. During surgery, chemotherapy, and doctor's visits, she was optimistic about the future. I wanted to stop when she passed away and take time to grieve, but I realized that the military doesn't slow down, especially during times of war. We were both in the Army now, and we had to stay in pace with the events of the world. What I learned from this is no matter what happens in life, time marches on, and it's important to put on your running shoes and keep going.

Jerry started training with the troops in his command on a rigorous schedule every day of the week. We kept our routine of getting up every morning and working out at the gym or going for a run, and then I made breakfast and Jerry went to work. Knowing my husband was training to fight in a war was stressful. Driving through the gates at Fort Hood filled me with anxiety. It was stressful seeing all the tanks, helicopters, and artillery ready to go to war. My eyes teared up knowing all the soldiers I saw were going to fight in a war and many would sustain serious injuries and be disabled for life or not come home. I spent days going through the many boxes that came up to my chest. I continued going through everything and throwing out anything that had been crumbled or stained. Since his moves were so frequent, Jerry didn't have the luxury of time to organize his possessions into save, donate, or trash piles. Every time he moved, the boxes got bigger and filled with more years of stuff I had to sort through. I started every morning after our workout and didn't stop until he got home at night.

We got engaged on the move to Fort Hood, and now we had to figure out when to have our wedding. Not knowing what would happen after deployment, I thought the sooner the better. We both wanted a summer wedding, but with the busy training schedule and command of a unit at Fort Hood and Fort Carson, Colorado, we had to look at when he could take time off to get married. He had three days around January 31, 2004, which was a few months after we moved into our house. I started planning the wedding, and it seemed since he only had three days off, a location wedding was the best thing to do. We found a wedding chapel off the Vegas strip and decided to have them cater the wedding. We only had three months to plan everything.

The wedding

Flying to Las Vegas carrying a wedding dress was probably not unusual, but it was never what I thought I would be doing. We invited everyone but ended up with about 20 guests and family, which made it perfect. My mom and one of my friends helped me get ready and we went to the chapel, but the couple before us wasn't done yet. I stood for about an hour in heels and my wedding dress, waiting for our turn. I was freezing and my feet were numb.

When it was our turn, I went outside and it was really cold. The music started playing "Here Comes the Bride," but no bride was coming because I'd forgotten my bouquet. The wedding coordinator asked, "Where is your bouquet?" I said, "I don't know." She went back to the side room and got my bouquet. The music started again, and I walked in.

Seeing Jerry standing at the altar wearing his Army dress blues was the most exciting moment of my life. Even though we'd rehearsed the night before, I was nervous and shaking as my son walked me down the aisle. The minister began the ceremony, and when it was my turn for vows, I was ready to burst into tears. We exchanged vows, put the rings on, and were pronounced husband and wife. When the words "you may kiss the bride" were spoken, we enjoyed a long kiss.

Our reception was in the hall next door so we could walk there when everyone was inside waiting for our appearance. We took photos in the church before we went to the dinner. The menu was mostly things with meat and sauces. I requested shrimp, melon, and strawberries for my meal. Our cake was a carrot cake. I wanted the traditional cake cutting and feeding each other cake, but I hadn't eaten cake in years. When Jerry put the cake in my mouth, I didn't know what to do with it. People who knew I didn't eat cake were watching closely to see what I would do. I swallowed it, but one bite was enough. I was happy with my special meal.

The honeymoon had to be delayed until June due to a mission Jerry had to go on once we got home from three days off. I didn't know where he was going, but we would have no contact once he left. This would be another challenging, stressful time I would have to deal with.

At the most stressful times in life, exercise can be the best way to calm the nerves and bring some joy to life. This mission my new husband was going on would be the first time he would be gone and I wouldn't know where he was or even if he was safe. The routine I had of getting up early and going for a run and going to the gym was the best way for me to deal with the anxiety of being a military spouse.

After the 30-day mission concluded and Jerry returned home safe, we could plan our honeymoon. All I knew was that it was out of the country, and I had never been outside of the United States other than on a day trip to Mexico. The stress of this was not the same as him being gone with no communication. We would be together, and he had everything set up. All I knew was there was a beach involved, and that sounded wonderful to me. What didn't sound great was flying to another country and not being able to bring my own food.

Going through customs, they would ask if I brought any food. This was scary, and I tried not to let it get to me, but what did they consider food? A package of tuna, a sandwich for the plane, some fruit? I thought if I brought food to eat before we took off out of Miami, I could eat it before we landed and not have any problems. This was a solid plan. Being prepared was what I liked to be, but I didn't want to break any rules.

When we got to customs, they didn't ask me about food at all. While walking out on the tarmac to the small plane, it was very humid, and once inside, I started to feel claustrophobic. I had to fall back on my knowledge of breathing to relax and calm my mind. This is another time that living a positive healthy and active life kept my mind and body healthy. No one knows what is in the future. All we know is today. We must give it our all. No matter what life throws at us, we need to keep charging forward in a healthy, positive way.

Lake Austin
My aunt and uncle moved to Austin the same month I moved to

Fort Hood. We didn't have any organic food stores in Morgan's Point Resort or Belton, so I drove to Austin to Whole Foods once a week and met my aunt and uncle for lunch and grocery shopping. When Jerry was gone on a mission, I would spend the night with them and go to the lake and ride my bike and run. I learned how to row at Lake Austin, where I would go whenever Jerry was on a mission. Rowing around the lake was peaceful. I had to keep busy so I wouldn't worry about him and all the other soldiers in harm's way. I continued eating my vegetarian foods and exercising daily whether I was at home or in California visiting my son and mom.

Being in a new state with a war going on and my husband preparing to deploy was daunting. The challenge of overcoming fear and maintaining a normal life at this time was difficult. We never knew what was going to happen. Helicopters break down and even crash during training. Focusing on exercise and maintaining healthy eating habits helped get us through every day. During night flight training, we had to get up at midnight so Jerry could train the troops wearing night-vision goggles. I never was able to go back to sleep. I stayed up until it got light and went for a run or to the gym. Jerry would have to stay at work once the sun came up and finish out the day.

Going to war

The duty of a commander's wife is to prepare everyone in the command for their spouse to be deployed at any time. I can remember a Christmas luncheon with all the troops that ended with the roll call of those soldiers deploying. All paperwork, childcare, wills, and power of attorneys had to be taken care of in advance so when it was time to deploy, they left at a moment's notice. Jerry and I knew the announcements were coming but couldn't let anyone know. It was difficult sitting through a

Christmas meal knowing that the deployment announcement was coming afterwards.

When times are challenging and changing, it's important to have an outlet for your feelings and stress. Running and working out was the best thing for us to do until it was time for Jerry to deploy. We lived each day to the fullest and spent as much time together as we could. Jerry had been a soldier much longer than I was a military spouse and a commander's wife. He helped me with everything I needed to do as "The Commander's Wife."

Thinking about what holds people back in life made me think of challenging times in my own life and how I usually handled them the same way. The power of positive thinking, praying, saying my mantras, and focusing on a positive outcome helped me through hard times.

Planning meals to take on the go

It's easy to prepare healthy meals and snacks wherever you go by planning in advance. Make a big pot of thick-cut or steel-cut oatmeal with cinnamon and stevia leaf and add vanilla protein powder mixed with almond milk or water after it's cooked. Stir it well, eat what you want, and save the rest for the next day. Top the oats with slivered almonds and dried or fresh berries. If you have a microwave at work, you can heat it up or eat it cold. I make my oat bars with stevia leaf, cinnamon, and dried fruit. My oat bars have protein, healthy carbohydrates, and fiber. They have everything needed for a meal replacement. Plain Greek yogurt, seasoned tofu, fresh fruit, and veggies are good for snacks. For lunch, it's easy to bring leftovers from dinner the night before or make a sandwich with tuna, seasoned tofu, nitrate-free deli meat, chicken, or turkey breast. Add some lettuce, spinach, cucumber, and tomato to get more veggies in your meal.

Travelling by plane is an opportunity to bring your own food, and you can buy water from the airport once you get through the TSA checkpoint. Water is very important when flying to prevent dehydration. Money can be saved by bringing your own food and snacks instead of paying the high prices at the airport. I recommend not drinking alcohol when flying if it's available. It's dehydrating and also affects your thought processes. When flights change or get cancelled, you need to be alert.

When I travel, I bring a lunch bag with sandwiches made with chicken breast or seasoned tofu, Japanese yams, cut fruit, date pieces, slivered almonds, stevia, and cinnamon. If they serve oatmeal on the plane, I add my cinnamon and stevia leaf. Rice cakes and trail mix are convenient snacks when you travel. I buy two large bottles of water once I get through the TSA checkpoint.

Another idea is to cook chicken breasts a day before you travel and freeze them in a baggie. Pack them in your suitcase. The chicken will be thawed when you arrive at your location, and you can put them in a refrigerator at your hotel. Buy a salad and vegetables from a local store and make a chicken salad.

Staying in a hotel is much easier when you stay at one with a refrigerator and a stovetop, or one that has a complete stove. This makes it easy to prepare healthy meals at the hotel and saves money when you don't have every meal at a restaurant. There are many markets or even small mini-markets that have eggs, cereal, milk, oatmeal, salad, vegetables, chicken, baked seasoned tofu, and fish. You can always bring a loaf of frozen bread in your suitcase if you know the stores around your hotel don't carry 100% whole grain breads. I prefer Ezekiel Bread, which some stores don't carry. In some stores, it can be found in the frozen section. These few items can be used for breakfast, lunch, and dinner.

Free breakfast at the hotel

Many hotels have a free breakfast. This is not the time to eat as much as possible. This is the time to choose wisely because you can. When I stay at a hotel that has oatmeal, I add my protein powder, stevia, dates, and almonds. If the oatmeal comes in a package, choose the plain or original oatmeal. Flavored oatmeal is loaded with sugar. If you have hard-boiled eggs, eat one yolk and three whites. If you can, eat oatmeal without adding any protein powder because you're getting protein from the eggs. Adding extra protein when you're working out is a good idea if you don't feel stuffed after you eat.

When you eat, you should feel satisfied, not overly full. If you feel stuffed, you're eating too much, too fast, or both. Your size, being male or female, and how much you exercise, will determine how much you can eat. If you eat more calories than you burn, you will gain weight. If you eat too much at one sitting, what your body does not use will be stored as fat for later use. If you do this on a regular basis, you're guaranteed to gain weight if you don't do enough exercise to burn off the excess calories.

Eat more when you exercise

Many people can consume more calories if they're training hard for a race, doing heavy weightlifting, or are very active. The more muscle you have, the more calories you burn, even at rest. Running and other cardiovascular exercises burn a lot of calories. Running will help you build muscle in the legs and get lean. This is an advantage to running. It also creates a euphoric feeling due to the release of endorphins, called a runner's high.

Drink water

Drinking water is the most important thing you can do for your

144

body so you don't get dehydrated. If you're thirsty, you're already dehydrated. Water supports brain function and helps keep you feeling full. Many people mistake thirst for hunger because they aren't drinking enough water. Be sure to drink plenty of water during and after exercise. If you feel thirsty, you've waited too long to drink water.

Make drinking water another habit by always bringing a few bottles of water with you. Start by drinking a full glass of water the minute you roll out of bed in the morning and continue drinking water all day long. It's essential that you drink water while you're exercising, and after exercising. When you sweat, you lose fluids, and you need to replace those fluids by drinking water. Sports drinks that claim to replenish electrolytes may have a lot of sugar and other ingredients like HFXA and artificial color, and ingredients that aren't good for the body. Water is always the best way to replenish electrolytes. Paying more money for drinks that claim to replenish electrolytes may be giving you extra sugar, and artificial ingredients that you don't need in your body.

Water can be carried in a bag or camel pack when riding a bike, running, or exercising. It keeps my hands free and keeps me hydrated during my outdoor exercise. This is an easy way to drink water while riding my bike, keeps my hands on the handlebars, and keeps me from being distracted while riding in traffic. Not reaching for the water bottle keeps focus on exercise and the surroundings while on the road. Water bags that strap around the waist or shoulders are ideal for running, hiking, and biking so the hands are free.

It's dangerous to become dehydrated, and going more than 72 hours without water can cause death. The signs of dehydration are dry mouth, dark urine, constipation, inability to urinate, feeling lightheaded or dizzy, and foggy thinking. The kidneys flush out toxins from the body and help the body to function. Going long periods without drinking or not drinking enough water can severely damage the kidneys. Always drink plenty of water throughout the day.

Team sports or community center activities

Finding something you like to do may involve joining a team sport. There are many team sports like volleyball, baseball, tennis, racquetball, football, gymnastics, cheerleading, and dance classes. If you get motivated by joining team sports, find a team or even a running or walking group.

There are classes at the gym or the local community center. Community announcements are posted, many of them online, and they're free or very low cost. Try several different classes and sports until you find what you love to do on a daily basis. You can also do a combination of classes and sports. Team sports challenge you, as do hobbies or a job that expands your mind and skills.

Chapter 9: Obesity and Children

Being overweight has recently become accepted in our society to the point where all commercials, advertisements for sports clothing, and women's clothes have plus-size models. This sends a confusing message to children concerning obesity.

Obesity is an epidemic in America and has become worse over the years of the pandemic with the shutdowns and uncertainty and fear of getting sick. The facts show children are becoming obese at a younger age, which puts them at a high risk of type 2 diabetes, high blood pressure, heart disease, high cholesterol, and even cancer.

Children are following unhealthy eating examples at home, or they are watching television where the food manufacturers target them with their unhealthy products. When children become obese, they're at risk for all of the problems adults have when they're overweight. This is a serious problem because many of these children grow up to be morbidly obese adults unless they're taught how to eat a healthy diet.

By teaching children to eat the right foods and leading by example, they can grow and prosper as healthy adults. It's terrible to put a child on a diet, and it's unnecessary if you teach them at an early age how to make good food choices. Meals that contain whole foods in their natural states like fruits and vegetables, 100% whole grains, and lean proteins give them everything they need to stay healthy. They don't need junk foods, candy, donuts, or cereals that are high in sugar.

By giving your children healthy food from the beginning of their lives, they'll learn what food tastes like and how to make healthy choices when they're away from home. It doesn't mean they have to avoid a treat like frozen yogurt or ice cream for special occasions.

Eating sugary desserts every day leads to sugar cravings because of the lack of nutrition and fiber. I see kids that eat a small portion of food so they "save room for dessert." The only dessert should be fruit, a smoothie, plain yogurt with fresh berries, or Tracy's Healthy Oat Bars.

If you give your children healthy food and healthy snacks, they will not crave sugar and they will not be drawn into the scheme of the manufacturers of junk foods who target children.

Children need to be outside having fun riding bikes, roller skating, playing at the park, and playing sports. Children who sit in front of the computer screen or television for just one hour a day are very likely to be watching all the commercials that target children and promote unhealthy cereals, candy, and junk foods.

The more time children spend doing homework, reading, writing, playing sports, riding a bike, skating, running, and being active, the less time they'll spend in front of the TV or computer being preyed upon by advertisers who market junk foods and sugary drinks that cause weight gain. Teach your children to eat healthy foods and stay active so they can live a long, healthy life.

Internet and social media

The internet and social media create many problems that affect children, and one that's very common is online bullying and body shaming. It is very common for children and teens to use social media to attack other kids and make hurtful comments about their weight, how they look, and who they associate with. This is not new other than the changes in technology.

Before the term body shaming became popular, high fashion models were being criticized for being too thin. In 2004, the Olsen twins were being interviewed on *The Oprah Winfrey Show*, and she asked them what size they were. They were only teenagers at the time and were not expecting an ignorant personal question like this. The audience laughed, and the twins were obviously uncomfortable being put in a terrible position on live television. Oprah never apologized for her public bullying and body shaming. This type of public humiliation is very harmful to children and teenagers, especially girls.

Models and others in the public eye were scrutinized for their weight and even told they couldn't work unless they gained weight. Plus-size models started being featured in magazines and on television. There was an overabundance of these types of models that exceeded the market demand. The next trend was to tell everyone to love their body no matter what. Social acceptance is important, but is celebrating being overweight good for young girls? The reality is that it is just as important to maintain a healthy body weight. It's not good to be too thin or overweight, as there's a healthy place in the middle. The goal is to be physically fit by taking care of the only body you have. Helping people learn what foods they should eat and how they can stay healthy throughout life is my mission in writing my books and blogs.

Outdoor activities

There are many things to do in the great outdoors to get into a healthy state of mind and to lose those extra pounds gained from being sedentary. Start with a morning routine of taking a run, walk, or bike ride. Being outside gives you a feeling of freedom and a chance to get some vitamin D from the sun. There are many places to go, and some can be right outside your front door. Look for a quiet street that has little traffic or a nature trail where you can take the family. Exercising outside will make everyone feel good.

Parks are great places to take the family for a day of fun in the sun. Playground equipment is useful for learning hand-eye coordination, and the swings are fun at any age. Kids love to play, swing, climb, and be with other children. The park is a place to meet friends and build new relationships. Parks are also nice places to have lunch. Be sure to bring plenty of water to stay hydrated.

On an open field, you can play soccer, football, baseball, and softball, which all improve eye, hand, and foot coordination. This very important part of a child's development is also fun for the whole family.

Swimming is something everyone can enjoy. Many communities have swimming pools, and many parks have public pools. Swimming is an excellent exercise, and everyone should know how to swim. If you don't know how to swim, this is the perfect time to take swimming lessons. Babies as young as six months old can learn to float. Their high fat content makes it easy for them to learn. Children can start taking lessons with a parent at age one. Children can learn to hold their breath underwater and roll over and float. They can also learn how to get to the side of the pool. Survival skills are very important, especially for children aged one through four.

Whatever you decide to do for exercise, make getting outside a habit that you do every day. Try new activities, learn new skills, and experience something that you've never done before. The most important thing is to get your body moving and have fun doing it.

Healthy parents and children

When I started my first business in the early eighties, I had to work a lot of hours. I didn't have time to exercise every day or go to the beach like I did when I was younger. My job was physical and very difficult. I taped exercise shows to do at night when I got home. I worked so many hours that I didn't have time to do the exercise for myself. I had my son to take care of, and he loved to play sports, fly kites, run, and play at the park and beach. Those activities with him were my only exercise many days, and it was fun teaching him how to play sports and watching him grow and mature into an athletic, confident young man.

My first aerobics lesson was at home, watching it on television. The first time I went to a class was in 1992. Going to a class was a lot more fun than doing a television class. I was reminded of my days playing sports because I had a group of people around me. I had spent many years doing things alone or with my son. I taught him to play baseball, basketball, football, volleyball, racquetball, and soccer. I also taught him to ride a bike, roller skate, swim, and bodysurf. Teaching him all these things made him athletic, which kept him active and busy. We never sat in the house playing video games or watching television, and were always outside together doing activities.

Years of working so hard and so many hours gave me the money to take care of my son, but as he got older, I decided to pick him up from school and let him do his homework, then we would go get something to eat and talk before his practice.

I decided to get a cell phone, which was large compared to

phones now, so I could stay at practice with my son and run around the field or up and down the stairs to get some exercise and watch him with the team. I always went to every game my son had, even though the cell phone didn't work well when I was at his games. It was a really hard time in my life, but I had to put my son's needs first and work as much as I could to support him. There are many ways to fit exercise into your day, and I learned how to do this as a single mother running my own business.

For people who have lunch breaks, it's easy to fit a workout in. Go to the gym in the morning and go for a walk or a run at lunch. Skip lunch and go to the gym. Eat lunch when you get done working out. There are so many benefits to exercising, and getting a workout will make you look and feel fantastic. It's never too late to start an exercise program. Consult your doctor if you have any health issues or concerns.

There are many challenges in life and many things we all must do each day, but one thing is the same for all of us. We all have 24 hours in the day, and we must use them wisely. One of the best ways to increase the available time in your day is to stock your refrigerator and pantry with healthy meals and snacks.

When you have healthy foods on hand, it's easier for you to make meals at home instead of running out for fast food. Fast food is not fast when you have to get in the car and drive somewhere and wait for your meal, then drive home to eat. It costs a lot of money and it's full of artificial ingredients, fat, sugar, and high-fructose corn syrup.

When you have food that is good for you and your children at home, they can help you prepare healthy meals and learn how to make healthy food choices.

Teaching children to cook and clean the kitchen is something they can use throughout life. Teaching your kids to make healthy food choices when they're young will make life easier and healthier when they're grown.

Healthy kids

Many diseases have a direct correlation to eating unhealthy foods that are high in fat, sugar, artificial colors, flavors, and preservatives. Processed meats, processed foods, red meat, and foods void of nutrition should be eliminated from meals and snacks. The body is designed to use foods in their natural state, not artificial foods. Protein, carbohydrates, and healthy fats are vital for a healthy mind and body. Due to eating foods high in sugar and fat and low in nutrition, the body is left without the nutrients it needs to thrive. Eating processed foods, high-calorie foods, and a low-fiber diet leads to overeating, weight gain, obesity, diabetes, high blood pressure, high cholesterol, and many types of cancer. These diseases are now being seen in children, which used to only be seen in adults. My son has three daughters and is teaching them to eat healthy foods and stay active.

When my granddaughters come to my house, I always make their favorite meals and let them help me prepare them. Children love to help, and they can do everything from washing fruits and vegetables to cutting them when assisted by an adult. This teaches them how to use sharp knives and how to prepare meals. Time is much better spent together than driving to get fast food. They know I don't eat fast food and they never ask for it because they love the food I cook, especially when we prepare it together. Children as young as two-and-a-half years old can tear lettuce and put it in a salad bowl. They can do more complex tasks as they grow, and you can teach them at different stages of their lives. My granddaughters help me the same way my son helped when he was little. Learning good habits that last a lifetime makes all the difference in their lives and the lives of parents and grandparents.

Exercise is so important to everyone and is something that can be done as a family. Take your kids on a walk, a hike, a bike ride, or roller skating. Don't let them sit around the house and stare at a screen playing games. These games are addictive, and they replace the social interaction and exercise the children need daily. Walk them to school and keep them active. Teach them about food, how many calories are in what they eat, and how much exercise it takes to burn off those calories. Teach them to make healthy food choices even when you aren't around. Make healthy eating and exercise a priority.

Plant a garden with your children and let them be involved in growing and caring for the plants. When the vegetables are ready, they can pick them and learn how to cook them. This is a way to get your children involved, active, and making smart food choices. If your school doesn't have a garden, suggest that they start growing one.

Advocate for healthy meals to be served in the cafeteria so your kids can have a healthy hot meal at school. If this is not possible, make sure you prepare and provide them with a healthy breakfast and a healthy lunch. Avoid prepared meals like Lunchables, which are processed and loaded with salt, sugar, and very few nutrients. They are not a good choice for lunch for anyone. You're better off sending hard-boiled eggs and low-fat string cheese, fresh fruit, and plain Greek yogurt. Make sure your yogurt is of good quality, and if it's flavored, make sure it's actual fruit and not artificial flavoring.

Tuna makes a healthy sandwich, or teriyaki tofu on Alvarado Street or Ezekiel Bread. Nitrate-free turkey breast or lean nitrate-free beef or ham is also good, along with a slice of tomato and lettuce. A small salad goes well with a sandwich. Anything is better than processed or fast foods. You owe it to your children to eat healthily and exercise daily so you'll be around to see them grow up, and you owe it to them to teach them to eat healthily and exercise daily.

You are responsible for your children 100% of the time. Don't rely on the school to provide healthy meals. As a parent, it is your responsibility to make sure your children are eating a healthy lunch made with love. For parents that are overweight, it's time to take charge of your life and start my healthy eating plan. It doesn't take any more time or money to eat healthy. You'll find you spend less time and money eating healthy and exercising than you will when driving to get fast food. The diseases associated with obesity can be avoided by eating healthy and exercising daily.

When creating a budget for the month, compare the costs of organic versus non-organic. It may be a few more cents per pound, but if you cut out the junk foods and fast foods, you will realize you have money that you were spending on things that aren't good for you, including tobacco and alcohol, that can be spent on your food budget. Cut out the fancy coffee, sugary snacks, and extra gasoline that you use to run out for fast food and use it toward your healthy eating plan. This will be the best money you ever saved. Realize that you can afford to eat healthy and you CANNOT afford to keep eating junk foods. By taking care of yourself and your family, you are making an investment in your family's long, healthy future.

When my granddaughter Isabella was a baby, I wanted to make healthy snacks for her, so I created my oatmeal bars with no sugar, oil, butter, or artificial ingredients. To this day, all three of my granddaughters love to eat my oat bars. I taught them how to make my oat bars so they can make them with me. They love to help me make banana bread and date nut bread using the healthy recipes I created. Teaching them to eat healthy foods at a young age has really helped them understand the importance of eating a healthy diet. They all know how I eat, and they want to be like their Meme. They call me Meme, which is the name Isabella gave me when she was a baby.

All my granddaughters love salmon and broccoli, which was their first solid meal. They also love brown rice. As a toddler, Isabella loved to go to the park in Los Gatos, which had a playground with swings and slides, a train, a fighter jet to climb on, and a carousel. After we played, we went to Whole Foods, which was close to the park. She called it the Princess Castle because the roof was shaped like a castle. We would get brown rice sushi, and she would have the sushi rice (brown rice), hearts of palm, and tofu. We did this during the first four years of her life, and it's still one of our favorite memories. Papa would take her to the flowers outside and teach her the colors.

Another fun memory of being in San Jose was taking our granddaughter to the farmer's market. We taught her about fruit and vegetables and how to pick the best ones. She loved to put the fruit and vegetables into the bag as Papa held it open. The bookstore was at the end of the block, and we always went in and looked at the books and bought books to read when we got back to their house. When Alexandra was born four years later, we had two granddaughters to do these fun things with, and she loved it as much as her sister.

Exercise is a very important part of life for children and should be started at a very young age. The city had "Mommy and Me" classes for children to interact with each other, and we started them with Isabella at a few months old. Her mother was working at the time, which gave me time to spend with Isabella, and I made the most of it. There were many parks to explore libraries, bookstores, and fun places to go.

I would take Isabella to my hotel to spend the night, and everyone at the hotel would gush over her and tell me how beautiful she was and how smart. Her first word was "Dada," her second "Mama," her third was "Papa," and then "Meme" and "hotel." When you're little, everything is so big and fascinating. All we had to do was take a walk around the hotel, and she was fascinated by everything. She found things that I never noticed, like flowers and seats in the halls, and stairwells with hiding places. In the morning, we went downstairs for breakfast and brought it up to our room to eat, then went to explore the hotel. This got her in the habit of exercising after breakfast. We got our exercise walking the halls and letting her explore.

My granddaughters love to run, play tag, ride bikes, hike, go on nature walks, swim, play soccer, and jump on their trampoline. One of their favorite games has always been playing zombie tag at the park with their Papa. Now that our youngest granddaughter, Evangelina, is five years old, she loves to run, play at the park, climb the rock wall, and swing on the monkey bars. She joined her sisters on the swim team this year and was also on the soccer team.

One of the things we love to do together is dance and exercise party, where each person gets a turn to pick the exercise we will all do. Isabella and Alexandra have taken some gymnastic classes, so they add some roundoffs, walkovers, and cartwheels. We bought them some gymnastic mats for Christmas that are long and soft so they can practice their gymnastics at home. It is fun watching them do the moves they learned in gymnastics. There are also kid's dance and exercise classes online or streaming that are good for getting exercise indoors on a cold or rainy day.

Leading by example is one of the best things you can do for children and teens because if they see you eating healthy foods and getting daily exercise, they'll want to do the same. Find fun family activities that everyone can do together like biking, hiking, skating, basketball, baseball, or just play catch. There are many ways to do fun family exercise, and it's important to teach your children how to stay healthy.

When it comes to meals, make every meal and snack packed full of vitamins by adding healthy vegetables, fruits, 100% whole grains, and beans. Create meals with a variety of colors to ensure you're getting a variety of vitamins from your food. You can always add fruits and vegetables as a side dish to your main dish. If you're making pasta, use 100% whole grain, and add a salad with garbanzo beans, kidney beans, hearts of palm, red cabbage, spinach, and strawberries. All the color means you're getting a variety of vitamins along with vital fiber. Fiber aids in digestion and helps keep you feeling full, and the complex carbohydrates provide energy to get through school, activities, and work.

Isabella
The day I found out my son was going to be a father and I was going to be a grandmother, I was thrilled. When I found out he was having a girl, I was ecstatic. Coming from a family where I had three brothers and then had a son, I was excited to have another girl in the family. The thoughts of buying pink clothes and baby dolls warmed my heart. I started thinking about all the things we could do together and what I could teach her. The night she was born was the greatest night of my life, not including having my son.

A few days later in December, our precious granddaughter made her appearance in the world, and I was there waiting for her. She was so beautiful and perfect, with a full head of hair just like her daddy when he was born. My heart was filled with tremendous joy watching her and holding her little hand. She was born late at night, but I wanted to stay until the nurses said it was time to go.

All I wanted was for it to be morning so I could go back to the hospital and see beautiful Isabella.

During the first month of Isabella's life, I was with her every day and loved every moment of it. I flew out to see her every other month and stayed in a nearby hotel. The time I got to spend with Isabella helped me bond with her, and it gave her parents a break so they could do things they needed to do without taking the baby with them. I was already working on healthy recipes to make for Isabella once she was able to eat solid food. My oat bars were the first recipe I created especially for Isabella with no sugar or butter, just healthy ingredients. Once she was old enough to eat my oat bars, they were an instant hit. They were so good that I decided to make them part of my diet also. My job was to teach Isabella how to eat healthy foods and take her to farmer's markets and parks so we could have fun while learning about healthy foods.

Isabella was three months old when Jerry returned home from Afghanistan. We flew out to California so he could meet his granddaughter. He brought car magazines and taught her how to flip the pages as he read stories about the cars. This was truly a special time. We developed a very strong bond with our Isabella. She loved the sound of her Papa's voice and always wanted him to read to her. She developed a great love for stories and reading.

Isabella, my oldest granddaughter, has spent the most time with us. She always asks for tofu, salmon, brown rice, and broccoli and she also loves Ezekiel Bread with veggie cheese, fresh fruit, and garbanzo beans. She is beautiful, healthy girl, and full of life. She has played softball, soccer and taken gymnastics, trampoline, tennis, and swim classes. She was on swim team and now plays soccer. She has my son's outgoing personality and love for people. She loves being active and being creative.

The recommendations from Isabella are to eat healthy foods

like tofu, garbanzo beans, hearts of palm, salads, broccoli and salmon, chicken breast and cauliflower, and lots of fruits. She loves Ezekiel sesame bread with veggie cheese, and Amy's organic bean and rice burritos. Another tip from Isabella is not to eat junk food and sugary snacks and drinks with sugar and caffeine.

The important lessons Isabella learned from me about healthy eating are still with her today. As a young teen, she still loves to eat healthy foods. Therefore, I decided to put her recommendations for healthy eating in this book.

Isabella's advice for kids

For breakfast, Ezekiel sesame bread is great toasted with veggie cheese on it. Nature's Path makes some healthy dry cereals with whole grains, and they are low in sugar. They're good with low-fat milk or unsweetened vanilla almond milk. I love to make smoothies with different fruits and have them for breakfast.

Oatmeal is also good to have for breakfast, and you can add fresh fruits and berries to give it more flavor and vitamins. Low-fat Greek yogurt with berries and stevia is also good for breakfast and as a snack between meals or after school. It's also a good and healthy dessert to have after dinner.

Amy's bean and rice organic burritos are on a 100% whole-wheat shell. They come frozen and can be cooked in the microwave in just a few minutes. They're good for you and they taste great. Amy's salsa or Muir Glen salsa is also great on the burrito.

Peanut butter or almond butter with jelly, Simple Fruit or similar fruit spread on a sandwich on 100% whole grain bread such as Ezekiel Bread, tossed salad, fresh fruit and water or low-fat milk is also a healthy lunch.

For dinner, one of my favorite things has always been salmon and broccoli with brown rice. I also love my dad's grilled chicken breast and vegetables like broccoli, cauliflower, peas, and corn on the cob. Since I'm allowed to cook now, I make pasta with sauce and garlic bread with a salad.

Meme created an oat bar recipe for me when I was a little girl, and I still love them for a snack or with lunch. Hearts of palms are great to snack on and so are garbanzo beans. I love rice cakes, dried fruit, plain yogurt, low or nonfat, with fresh berries and stevia leaf mixed in. Fresh fruit and melon are tasty, and I also like 100% whole-grain crackers with low-fat string cheese.

Lunch is a great time for a sandwich with tofu, turkey, or ham with cheese on wheat bread, peanut butter and jelly, cheese sandwich, wheat toast with avocado, or an Amy's bean and rice burrito. I love teriyaki tofu on Ezekiel sesame bread with dijon mustard. I also love Ezekiel sesame bread with veggie cheese. Low-fat milk is what I usually have with meals, and I drink water.

Dinner foods are salmon and broccoli, brown rice, cauliflower, chicken breast, asparagus, green beans, mixed vegetables, potatoes, yams, squash, and peas. I always love brown rice sushi with garbanzo beans and watermelon and cantaloupe. Meme and Papa always took me to Whole Foods for lunch and let me choose what I wanted from the salad bar. Now I also like brown rice California rolls.

It is very important to eat a balanced meal that has fruits such as berries, melon, apples, and any other fruit. Eating vegetables is very important and fish, chicken, and beef are good for protein.

Tossed salad is lettuce, spinach, and a few whole-grain croutons with low-fat Italian dressing or vinegar. You can have chicken, salmon, or any type of fish or tofu with your salad. Always eat vegetables with your meal so you get a lot of vitamins and protein. It is important to eat vegetables and 100% whole grains so you get a variety of vitamins and get fiber in your meals.

Exercise is very important to stay healthy, and I love to take gymnastics, swim, ride bikes, skate, and do things with my friends. For today, we're going to do 20 pushups, 15 sit-ups, 20 crunches, 30 mountain climbers. We jump rope, run laps, and play field hockey.

Group activities include a partner work dance like acrobatic dance, where you combine gymnastics and dancing moves. They can be done in a group or with a partner.

Soccer is another good activity that gets your heart rate up and helps you burn calories. After lunch is a good time to do some exercise and burn off the calories you ate. It's good for kids to have activities after lunch so they can play before they return to the classroom and concentrate on learning.

Our P.E. teacher has a special activity for Grandparents' Day. The grandparents can walk and talk while walking around the track. They can come to their grandchildren's class and see what subjects they're working on and look at their work.

Alexandra

When Alexandra was six years old, she told me what she wanted to tell kids to eat, and I wrote it down for her. She loves to help me cook meals, make salads, and bake oat bars, banana bread, and date bread. When it's time to go out and play, she's the first one out the door. She has a lot of energy and does as much as she can in a day. She joined the swim team this year and didn't know all of the strokes, but she spent a lot of time with her Papa and me in the pool at the hotel and learned to swim. She worked hard at practice and won a lot of ribbons from the swim team. She is very proud of her accomplishments, and we are too.

Alexandra is now nine years old, and she continues to love to eat healthy food and exercise. She loves taking gymnastics, soccer, tennis, and swim lessons. This year, she was on a year-round swim team and did very well. Alexandra loves to color and play games and cards with us, and she loves to read. She's an excellent student and has a lot of friends. She also enjoys helping around the house and doing yard work with her dad. She is a wonderful granddaughter, and we love spending time with her.

Alexandra's advice for kids
Eat lots of fresh fruit and vegetables. Eat a balanced meal with 100% whole grains and lean protein. Make sure to eat a variety of vegetables and fruits like apples, cherries, grapes, mangos, and pears along with broccoli, spinach, cauliflower, cabbage, green beans, asparagus, corn, peas, and carrots.

A good meal for breakfast is oatmeal. Eat whole fruit instead of drinking juice, and drink a lot of water. For lunch, try tofu on 100% whole grain bread like Ezekiel Bread or a tortilla with lettuce, low-fat cheese or cottage cheese, low-fat vegetarian refried or black beans, and salsa. For dinner, grill some chicken breasts, carrots, corn, and broccoli, and drink more water. Another dinner or lunch can be sushi made with brown rice. Kids like California rolls, and adults love tuna and avocado rolls. You can have a little treat like a little sucker made with natural ingredients.

Healthy snacks can be fruit by itself or with plain yogurt, with berries and a little stevia. A smoothie made with low-fat milk, apple juice, fresh or frozen strawberries, mango, blackberries, and a scoop of Juice Plus for a healthy protein and carbohydrate drink. Organic gummy snacks that are low in sugar and made with natural ingredients are better than the ones that have artificial ingredient colors and flavoring. Make homemade ice cream with low-fat milk and Greek yogurt sweetened with stevia and natural vanilla bean for flavor. Homemade banana bread and other low-fat baked goods made with healthy ingredients are also tasty options.

It's important to eat healthy food and drink a lot of water so you won't get fat. Don't drink soda, because it will rot your teeth and has a lot of sugar and calories.

Evangelina

Evangelina is my youngest granddaughter, and she always tries to keep up with her older sisters. From the time she was born, she's been following them around, trying to do everything they do, and she has no fear. She'll jump in the pool, jump off a wall, and meet any challenge. She has a mind of her own. She always wants to play Legos, do yoga, exercise, and walk to the park to play. She loves to play cards and games, and we have a wonderful time playing with all our granddaughters.

Evangelina loves to eat teriyaki-baked tofu, just like her sisters, which I introduced them to when they were toddlers. She also loves Amy's bean and rice burritos. When we go to the park, I bring my oatmeal bars, tofu, fruit, and gummies. They all love bringing that same snack to the park to this day.

Evangelina has some things she likes to eat that her sisters don't eat, like eggs. She likes them scrambled and wants pepper on them. She likes to eat yogurt with bananas or berries, smoothies with fruit, and chips and salsa. She likes rice cakes just like her sisters, and she loves to play at the park and go for walks.

It's very rewarding having an influence in my granddaughters' lives and leading by example where they eat the healthy meals I prepare and reflect my morals and values. At home, my son makes healthy meals for the girls. Being consistent helps create a habit of healthy eating. Eliminate sugar and junk foods that are full of artificial ingredients and processed to the point they lack nutrition and fiber. The burst of energy from sugar leads to a spike in blood sugar, followed by a crash in blood sugar, which leads to cravings for more sugar.

Junk foods are loaded with high-fructose corn syrup and other sugars, artificial flavors, colors and ingredients, sodium, and MSG, which is unhealthy for the body and creates cravings for more junk food. This leads to weight gain, obesity, high cholesterol, high blood pressure, heart disease, and even cancer when consumed on a regular basis. By avoiding junk foods, processed foods, and anything with artificial ingredients, you're giving the body what it needs to grow healthy and stay healthy.

Children are exposed to so much sugar, junk foods, fast foods, artificial sweeteners, and preservatives, along with excess hormones in our food supply. There are also toxins in our shampoos, soaps, and household cleaning products. Parabens are chemicals that are known to create xenoestrogens and can mimic estrogen and contribute to early puberty. This is something that has greatly increased over the past 10 years.

One in three kids is obese, and children are developing diseases that only adults used to have. The culprits are in our food supply and our homes. The Food and Drug Administration (FDA) allows hormones to be used in our food supply such as estradiol, estriol, testosterone, growth hormone, and progesterone. These hormones wreak havoc on our bodies and cause children to go into early puberty.

Fast foods and junk foods are causing our children to become obese, where they can develop high blood pressure, high cholesterol, type 2 diabetes, and cancer. Studies have shown the rate of breast cancer increases with the onset of early puberty and causes the bones to not develop correctly. Puberty should not begin until age 13 or 14. Children are going into precocious puberty, which is going into puberty at an early age before they're ready. Some girls as young as seven years old are developing breasts, which is one of the signs of early puberty. About a year after this, girls will start menstruating, which is challenging in so many ways for a girl at such a young age when they're not emotionally ready.

There are many things you can do to prevent early puberty, and eating a healthy diet full of fresh organic fruits and vegetables and lean organic proteins that don't have any hormones added will help a lot. Stay away from preservatives, additives, and chemicals that have long names. If you can't pronounce the ingredient, you and your children should not eat it. Pesticides mimic hormones and should be avoided by eating an organic diet and buying produce from a local farmer's market. Buy organic lotions and shampoo, or at least make sure your products don't contain parabens. Use natural cleaners like vinegar, lemon juice, and baking soda.

Dr. Jennifer Landa of BodyLogicMD of Orlando recommends preventing precocious puberty by doing the following:

1. Go green. Use all-organic produce, shop at farmer's markets, and use natural cleaners like baking soda, lemon juice, and vinegar.
2. Become a label reader and avoid products with long words ending with "eth." Avoid products that have parabens, sodium lauryl or lauretha sulfite, and triclosan and triethanolamine, or TEA.
3. Exercise daily by walking with your family, playing sports, jumping rope, or going to the park to play tag. Encouraging physical exercise helps child weight management and will further reduce their exposure to hormones.

Eating healthy is the most important thing you can do for yourself and your children. Make sure that you're doing all you can to stay healthy so you can be around to take care of your children, and make sure they stay healthy and maintain a healthy weight.

In 2016, the FDA issued a rule that many over the counter products that contain triclosan were potentially harmful. Antibacterial active ingredients including triclosan and triclocarban can no longer be added to products marketed to consumers. These products include liquid soaps, liquid and foam hand gel, hand soap, bar soap, and body washes. Triclosan is also added to certain clothes, cookware, furniture, and toys to reduce and prevent bacterial contamination, but these are not regulated by the FDA. The study has raised questions about whether triclosan is hazardous to human health. Researchers found triclosan alters hormone regulators in animals and contributes to the development of antibiotic-resistant germs and might be harmful to the immune system.

A study designed to test the amount of triclosan exposure took urine samples from adults and children in 2008 and found that 75% contained triclosan in their urine. Triclosan is not an essential ingredient. It may help prevent gingivitis when added to toothpaste, but there is no evidence that antibacterial soaps and bath wash are more effective than regular soap in preventing illness or the spread of certain diseases, according to the FDA. Make sure your children are using natural products, and avoid BPA plastics. Never heat up food or put hot food in a plastic container or bag. Cleaning with vinegar, lemon juice, and baking soda is very cheap and much safer for your family. Avoid products that are scented, and look for all-natural ingredients. This will help keep your children and you from being exposed to dangerous chemicals that cause illness and hormone problems.

One of the things that kids are consuming that is terrible for them is the yellow-orange powder on chips and macaroni and cheese. This powdery substance reportedly causes problems with the thyroid and hormonal system. You hear many people saying they ate a whole bag of chips, and that they're addicting. The chemicals in many products and fast foods are addicting. They make you eat more, and this is profitable for the manufacturers.

It's bad for you and your children because along with all the chemicals that disrupt your hormonal system, they also cause obesity. Talk to your children and teach them portion control, and teach them what is healthy and what they need to avoid. It is essential for us to all work together to eliminate diseases and other problems caused by eating an unhealthy diet and being exposed to chemicals that are known to cause cancer and disrupt your normal hormonal system. If you stay aware and act now to make these important changes, you can save your children and yourself a lot of heartache and money by implementing a healthy eating plan and eliminating as many chemicals as you can from your diet and your surroundings.

Healthy for life

My goal is to give you creative ways to exercise regardless of where you are or what shape you're in. It's important to take at least one hour a day to do some form of exercise. Running, brisk walking, biking, and lifting weights are all effective forms of exercise. Moving your body gets your heart pumping and your blood flowing. Many people are living into their 90s and even more beyond the century point, because they do physical activity and eat healthy foods. They take time to enjoy life and have fun with friends and family. Many people are still working into their 90s, doing things that use the brain to stay mentally sharp. My father-in-law, Jerry Dwyer Sr., was doing his taxes, investing in the stock market, and helping his kids make wise investing decisions throughout his lifetime. He continued doing things that kept him thinking and moving his body until his very last days. He always said to look into the future and take good care of your health, and take time to put your feet up.

I used to take tap dancing classes when I was very little. My mom took me out when I was five years old, but I always missed it. As an adult, I joined an adult tap class at the community center, and I loved it. I was the youngest one in the class. I couldn't keep up with the ladies who were 20 years older than I was. They were great tap dancers and had a lot of energy. I went to the class after work every Tuesday and Thursday night from six to eight. We learned two dance numbers and performed at a dance recital at the park with all the other dancers from other classes. I took acting and vocal classes at a local community college just to stay active and involved, and I could schedule work around my classes. This was a huge source of pleasure and showed me that it's never too late to start or return to something you love.

Conclusion

Life is what you make of it, and how you spend every day is up to you. Choosing to be happy and healthy is one of the best decisions you will ever make. Don't waste time on anything negative, and don't sit around feeling sorry for yourself or making excuses for not doing things that you want to do. Find a way to accomplish all your goals, and live life to the fullest. Remember, life is not a dress rehearsal. This is your life, and you need to take full control and full advantage of every opportunity to enjoy each day and make the most out of every hour in the day.

Life is like running in a race. You will feel great, then tired, then have a burst of energy, and then feel great again. You never know when you're at the finish line of life. It's important to make every minute of every day count.

My health has always been important to me, and I always tried to take care of myself and everyone around me. I never took my health for granted. I always tried to do some form of exercise and eat healthy foods. At the least, I ate an apple every day and still do. My version of healthy has changed over the years since I was living under my mother's roof. I had to eat what she was making for dinner. We used to go to Lindberg Nutrition, which was a health food store with a little café area. I learned about yogurt, healthy foods to eat, and to stay away from sodas. We never had sodas at home, but we did drink them in the summer when we went camping. The rest of the time, we had milk, orange juice, or water. I loved when we had water delivered to our house and we could get spring water. It tasted so good! I still love spring water and drink it all day long. It is so important to remember the little things that make a big difference in your health. Drinking plenty of water is at the top of the list. Eat healthy foods in their natural state, and exercise daily. These are important to living a very healthy life.

Make a commitment to yourself to stay healthy for a lifetime. It's not something you do just for a special occasion. Eating healthy food and doing exercise daily is for life. Life is not a sprint; it's a marathon, and if you aren't physically fit and healthy, you may not make it to the finish line. Think of yourself as an athlete, whether you are or not. Think of every day as your training for the main event called life. Every workout, every meal, everything you do is leading up to the main event.

Don't forget the short races you must run before the marathon or the Ironman Triathlon (swimming, biking, and a marathon), which you use as training in a short distance run, bike, or swim. Life throws all sorts of curveballs your way, and you don't know what's ahead of you no matter how much you plan or how hard you try. But if you're physically fit and eating healthy, you'll be better equipped to handle whatever life sends your way. It's said that God doesn't give you more than you can handle. It's also said that what doesn't kill you makes you stronger. If you're prepared for the curveball and you train for the main event called life, you will succeed and get through whatever comes your way.

About the Author

Do you want to achieve a high level of fitness and overall great health in your life? You have the power within yourself to achieve all your goals. Tracy Dwyer is an author, nutritionist, and health and wellness expert who shared her knowledge in her book *Healthy Meals in Minutes*. She has dedicated her life to teaching people how to live a healthy lifestyle. Eating healthy meals and getting daily exercise is a great way to achieve all your future goals. In *Healthy Meals in Minutes*, Tracy shared her knowledge of what foods are the best to eat to stay healthy for life. In her new book, *Fit and Healthy Throughout Life*, she shares her voluminous knowledge detailing what it takes to stay healthy at any age through all of life's challenges.

Tracy attended Pepperdine University in Malibu and Loyola Marymount University, where she earned a Bachelor of Arts degree in Film and Television. She started two successful businesses, one in Los Angeles and one in San Jose, California. Tracy and her son, Justin, moved to San Jose, where she worked as a videographer for the news, special events, church services, city council meetings, and television programs. Tracy has been seen on camera in several television series such as *Nash Bridges* and the movie *Patch Adams*, as well as appearing in many local and national commercials.

Diagnosed with colon cancer at 36 years old, Tracy felt it was her calling to spread awareness and let everyone know that young people do get colon cancer. Becoming a member of Toastmasters International gave Tracy the experience she needed to become a motivational speaker and a spokesperson for the American Cancer Society, where she spoke about her experience with colon cancer and what steps she took to ensure she would never get cancer again. Tracy wrote and presented many public service announcements on television giving the warning signs of colon cancer, the number-two cause of death from cancer in both men and women. She is a lifetime practitioner and acolyte of nutrition and living a healthy happy life.

Tracy has studied nutrition and exercise for years and is taking classes to become a registered dietician. Her mission is to teach others how to make healthy eating and exercise a priority in their lives. It has been over 28 years since her unlikely diagnosis of colon cancer with no recurrence of cancer due to her healthy eating, exercise, and positive lifestyle.